Case Studies in Emergency Medicine

Volker Wenzel

Editor

Case Studies in Emergency Medicine

A Collection of Memorable Clinically Relevant Cases with Clinical Pearls

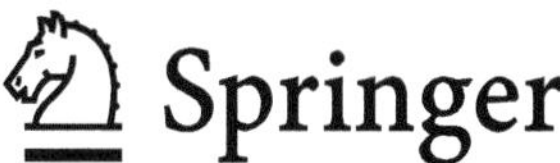

Editor
Volker Wenzel
Department of Anesthesiology
Intensive Care, Emergency Medicine
and Pain Therapy
Friedrichshafen Regional Medical Center
and Tettnang Hospital
Friedrichshafen, Baden-Württemberg
Germany

ISBN 978-3-662-67248-8   ISBN 978-3-662-67249-5   (eBook)
https://doi.org/10.1007/978-3-662-67249-5

This Springer imprint is published by the registered company Springer-Verlag GmbH, DE, part of Springer Nature.
The registered company address is: Heidelberger Platz 3, 14197 Berlin, Germany

Preface

There are experiences in emergency medicine everyday life which one does not forget for professional or human reasons. Unfortunately, colleagues from other regions can hardly learn from these extraordinary experiences, because they are usually only communicated in the immediate environment—they "usually" do not fit into a scientific article, "standard operating procedures" or even clinical guidelines. Despite missing this trigger threshold, these experiences illustrate that emergency medical care can not always be forced into templates of a guideline; this will regularly fail. Rather, the experiences described in this book show how important personal experience, clinical skills and wise assessment of complex situations by the emergency physician are in unpredictable situations in order to optimize the care of the emergency patients entrusted to us.

In the present book, authors with cumulatively several hundred years of experience in emergency medicine have described experiences that they will not forget. But it's not just real descriptions of extraordinary missions, but they also show the courage and sincerity of the authors to tell about their disappointments, fears and even their personal failure. Based on difficult situations, one can develop personally and professionally much better than if everything went well by chance—then one is patted on the shoulder by everyone. Each of us can become better personally, in the family and professionally; regardless of age, profession, rank or life experience. A prospective decision is much more difficult than retrospective assessment; hopefully this book will facilitate a fruitful discussion of difficult experiences and ultimately decisions in difficult situations.

All authors have written their book chapters in their spare time, on weekends or on vacation, for which I can not thank them enough; I am proud to work with them. Dr. Anna Krätz has helped my idea for this book at Springer Publishing house with good arguments to the "Go" and has driven the project continuously and always on schedule together with Axel Treiber. Dr. med. Dipl.-Päd. Martina Kahl-Scholz has excellently supervised all chapters as a lecturer.

As in emergency medicine, it is the team performance of many different people with very different talents that makes the decisive difference with this book— many heartfelt thanks to all of them! I would like to thank my wife Dr. Regina Wenzel and our daughters Katharina, Anna and Clara for their patience, support and love. You raise me up to more than I can be.

I am very pleased about constructive criticism of this book—science and thus clinical treatment strategies are always in flux and it is never too early to plan the next edition of this book (volker@wenzelcloud.com).

I wish you a lot of fun and excitement while reading!

Friedrichshafen   Prof. Dr. Volker Wenzel M.Sc., FERC
in fall 2023

Contents

Editor and Contributors

About the Editor

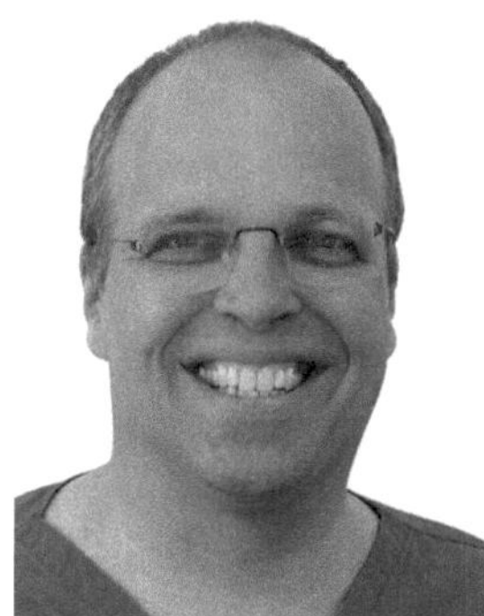

Prof. Dr. med. Volker Wenzel M.Sc. FERC is Chairman of the Department of Anesthesiology and Intensive Care Medicine, Emergency Medicine and Pain Therapy of Medical Campus Lake Constance-Friedrichshafen Regional Medical Center and Tettnang Hospital.

He is the author or co-author of more than 330 peer-reviewed articles and 40 book chapters, co-editor of two books and editor of the emergency medicine section of the journal "Die Anaesthesiologie". He is Courtesy Professor of Anesthesiology at the University of Florida in Gainesville, Florida, United States. He looks back with pride on the successful supervision of 44 M.D. and Ph.D. thesis.

Contributors

Prof. Dr. med. Hans-Richard Arntz is an internist and cardiologist; he has been working as a senior physician at the Department of Cardiology and Pulmology at the Free University Berlin Campus Benjamin-Franklin and later at the Charité University Medicine Berlin, Germany since 1987. For 24 years, he was the medical director of the Emergency Medical Service Helicopter Christoph 31 and the physician-manned ambulance 4205 in Berlin-Steglitz, as well as of the early defibrillation program in Berlin. He is the author of 141 peer-reviewed articles and 31 book chapters, as well as the initiator and coordinator of several large clinical multicenter studies.

Franziska Böhler is an intensive care nurse and worked for 13 years in an anesthesiological intensive care unit in Frankfurt, Germany and now as an anesthesiology nurse in outpatient surgery. She published the Spiegel Bestseller "I'm a nurse" in 2020 and is active on Instagram as "thefabulousfranzi", where she has 280,000 subscribers. She has been a jury member of the Queen Silvia Nursing Award since 2019 and has appeared on breakfast television, HR, Kölner Treff, among others.

Priv.-Doz. Dr. med. Jan Breckwoldt MME was between 1998 and 2012 senior physician in the Department of Anesthesiology and Intensive Care Medicine at Campus Benjamin Franklin University Hospital of the Berlin Charité University Medicine and responsible there for the emergency medical service. After completing a master's degree in "Medical Education", he was also teaching coordinator and member of the project management for the model degree programme Medicine of the Charité University Medicine in Berlin, Germany. From 2013 to 2017 he headed the study dean's office of the Medical Faculty of the University of Zurich; since 2018 he has been senior physician in the Institute of Anaesthesiology at the University Hospital in Zurich, Switzerland. In parallel to his scientific core area of resuscitation, he is committed to competency-based medical education, including EPAs.

Priv.-Doz. Dr. med. Hermann Brugger is vice head of the EURAC Institute for Alpine Emergency Medicine in Bolzano, South Tyrol, lecturer at the Medical University of Innsbruck, Austria, member of the International Commission for Alpine Emergency Medicine ICAR MEDCOM and mountain rescue physician, emergency physician and general practitioner in Bruneck, South Tyrol, Italy.

Prof. Dr. med. Dr. h.c. Bernd Domres was professor of surgery at the University Hospital Tübingen, Germany from 1980 to 2003. From 1985 to 1988 he headed the surgery department of the King Khaled Hospital in Hail / Saudi Arabia. His focus is on trauma and disaster medicine. Since 1975 he has been a physician in numerous disasters—including in Nigeria, Cambodia, Lebanon, Armenia, Congo, Iran, Turkey, Italy, Haiti, Chile and Pakistan. He is president of the German Institute for Disaster Medicine and the Foundation of the German Institute for Disaster Medicine. He was president of the German Society for Disaster Medicine and was awarded the Federal Cross of Merit first class in 2012.

Priv.-Doz. Dr. med. Martin Dünser is a senior physician in the Department of Anesthesiology and Surgical Intensive Care Medicine at the Kepler University Hospital Linz, Austria. After completing his training as a specialist in anaesthesia and intensive care, he worked at the Department of Intensive Care Medicine at the University Hospital in Bern, Switzerland, at the Paracelsus Medical University in Salzburg, Austria as well as at the University College of London Hospital and the London's Air Ambulance, both in London/United Kingdom. In addition to his scientific activities in the treatment of critically ill patients, he was chairman of the Section Trauma and Emergency Medicine and the Global Intensive Care Working Group of the European Society of Intensive Care Medicine ESICM. He has worked a total of two years in emergency and intensive care in Africa and Mongolia.

Bernd Fertig is a certified paramedic (SRK) and holds a B.Sc. in interdisciplinary emergency care and a M.Sc. in EMS management. Since January 2020, he has been a visiting professor at the Faculty of Medicine San Ferndando, the Universidad

Nacional Mayor San Fernando in Peru and the autonomous University Gabriel Renè Moreno in Santa Cruz de la Siera in Bolivia. Bernd Fertig is building a competence center for EMS and air rescue in Lima, Peru with the support of the German federal government. He is currently supporting the treatment of Covid19 patients with a German and Peruvian team. Training as a certified paramedic in Switzerland and Seattle Medic 1 in Seattle. He is a teacher in the EMS and is currently heading a master's program for medical directors in Peru and Bolivia. He is also setting up a professional emergency medical service training according to German standards in Peru and Bolivia.

Dr. med. Norman Hecker is a specialist in anesthesiology, emergency medicine and clinical acute and emergency medicine. He holds the qualifications of emergency physician, senior emergency physician, medical director of emergency medical services and tele-emergency physician. Since 2018, he has been Chief Physician of the Department of Acute and Emergency Medicine at the Protestant Hospital Gelsenkirchen, Chief Emergency Physician of the City of Gelsenkirchen and Site Manager of physician-manned ambulance 30-1 at the Gelsenkirchen-Horst site. He attended Medical School at the Universities of Cologne and Valetta (Malta). From 2007 to 2013, he was project manager for emergency medicine at the German Institute for Disaster Medicine in Tübingen. He was also part of international disaster missions several times. Furthermore, he has been leading the bilateral Sino-German Institute for Disaster and Emergency Medicine (SGIDEM) at Tongji Hospital in Wuhan (Huazhong University for Science and Technology, Hubei, People's Republic of China) of the Sino-German and German-Chinese Medical Societies since 2015. He is one of the Hanno Peter Honorary Laureates of the German Society for Disaster Medicine (2015), Graduate Visiting Professor of the oldest continuously operating university in the Americas (Universidad Nacional Mayor de San Marcos UNMSM, Lima, Peru) in the field of Emergency and Disaster Medicine, member of the Scientific Advisory Board of the German-Chinese Society of Medicine, Post-Graduate of Karolinska University in Stockholm, Sweden (Medical Response to Major Incidents) and on the User-Advisory Board of the EU Horizon 2020 project Nightingale.

Priv.-Doz. Dr. med. Peter Hilbert-Carius (DEAA) is a senior physician in the Department of Anesthesiology, Intensive Care and Emergency Medicine at the BG Trauma Hospital Bergmannstrost in Halle, Germany. He is medical director of the DRF air rescue station in Halle (Oppin) and spokesperson for the Trauma Network Saxony-Anhalt South.

Priv.-Doz. Dr. med. Björn Hossfeld is a senior physician in the Department of Anesthesiology and Intensive Care Medicine at the Federal Armed Forces Hospital in Ulm, Germany, as well as a Leading physician of the Emergency Medical Service Helicopter „Christoph 22" and leading EMS-physician for the district of Ulm / Alb-Donau. He took part in several overseas deployments of the German armed forces in Afghanistan, Kosovo, Libanon, Mali, Niger, and the Congo.

Dr. med. Peer G. Knacke was already active in the noncombattant service and during his Medical School time in the Emergency Medical service; after graduation, he worked for three years in surgery and pediatric surgery; since 1988 he has been working in anesthesia. He is senior physician in the Department of Anesthesia and Emergency Medicine at the AMEOS Hospital Eutin, Germany, medical director of the Emergency Medical Service Ostholstein, representative of the leading emergency physician group and medical director of the EMS Helicopter „Christoph 12". So far, he has carried out over 15,000 independent emergency medical service scene calls in ground and air rescue services.

Dr. med. Joachim Koppenberg is Chairman of the Department of Anesthesiology, Pain Therapy and Emergency Medicine in Engadin / Switzerland since 2004. For over 22 years he has continuously worked in ground-based emergency medical services and also in air rescue—first with DRF in Germany, then with ÖAMTC in Austria and now with REGA in Switzerland. He has been Lead Emergency Physician and Station Physician of the Alpine Rescue Switzerland. In addition to numerous publications in emergency medicine, he is also editor of the Psychrembel AINS, section editor of the journal "Der Notarzt" and co-editor of the German translations of the AHA resuscitation guidelines (BLS, ACLS, PALS). At the same time, he is course director of the AHA for ACLS courses. His other areas of interest and research focus on risk management and patient safety. He is also CEO of the Unterengadin Health Center in Switzerland.

Prof. Dr. med. Frank Marx is a board-certified physician in Anesthesiology and Intensive Care. He has been working in the emergency medical service at various locations since 1992. After his medical training, he led the Institute for Emergency Medicine at Duisburg Hospital in Germany until 1997. As medical director of the emergency medical service, he was with the Duisburg Fire Department and served also on the emergency medical service helicopter "Christoph 9" and various other emergency medical services. As part of the foreign disaster relief of Malteser International, he has been active in Africa, Asia and North America. He now teaches at the Health Department of the TH Mittelhessen in Gießen, Germany Emergency Medical Service Management.

Prof. Dr. med. Marc O. Maybauer EDIC, FCCP, FACC, FASE Studied medicine at the Justus Liebig University in Giessen, Germany. His dissertation (M.D.) and habilitation (Ph.D.) both engaged with the management of acute lung injury and ARDS. He is an internationally renowned physician who received training in anesthesiology at the University Hospitals of Mainz and Ulm, Germany, cardiac anesthesia and transesophageal echocardiography at the Oxford Heart Centre, Oxford, UK, and Critical Care Medicine at the University of Texas Medical Branch at Galveston, USA. He served as director of the ECMO services at Manchester Royal Infirmary, Manchester, UK and the Integris Baptist Medical Center in Oklahoma City, USA. He recently was appointed as Professor and Chief of Critical Care Medicine, Executive Director for the Critical Care Organization, and Program Director for Adult ECMO at the University of Florida College of Medicine in Gainesville, USA. In addition, Professor Maybauer is holding a professorship at the Philipps University in Marburg, Germany, and an honorary professorship at the University of Queensland in Brisbane, Australia. He is the author of more than 200 scientific publications and winner of numerous awards. Professor Maybauer is the editor of the textbook: "Extracorporeal Membrane Oxygenation – A Problem-Based Learning Approach" with Oxford University Press.

Dr. med. Martin Messelken is board certified in Anesthesiology with the additional designation of Intensive Care Medicine and Emergency Medicine. From 1980 to 2013 he was responsible for the emergency medical service in Alb-Fils-Hospital Göppingen (formerly Klinik am Eichert) and in the last years of his career he was working as a leading senior physician. From 2005 to 2013 he was also an emergency physician on the EMS helicopter "Christoph 51". The publication and further development of the Minimal Emergency Medical Data Set (MIND) goes back to his initiative. In 2010 he received the Rudolf Frey Award for Emergency Medicine in Germany. He has been involved in the establishment of the German Resuscitation Registry as a member of the Organizing Committee from the beginning.

Priv.-Doz. Dr. med. Urs Pietsch DESA/EDIC is a senior physician in the Department of Anesthesiology and Intensive Care at Kantonsspital St. Gallen, Switzerland and medical director of the Resuscitation and Simulation centre Rea2000 in St. Gallen. In addition to his many years of prehospital work as an emergency physician (Air Zermatt, Switzerland), he is scientifically involved in the fields of simulation, alpine rescue medicine and alpine helicopter rescue.

Dr. med. Luise Schnitzer is board-certified in Cardiology, Emergency Medicine and Psychotherapy. She has been working in the Department of Cardiology and Pulmology at the Free University Berlin, and later at the Charité University Medicine Berlin, Germany Campus Benjamin Franklin since 1980, has been an emergency physician at the Emergency Medical Service Helicopter "Christoph 31" and physician-manned ambulance 4205 in Berlin-Steglitz since 1987 and has been leading emergency physician since 2001. She has been working mainly in the emergency service since 1995.

Dr. med. Sylvi Thierbach after attending Medical School at the University of Hamburg, she was a resident at the Federal Armed Forces Hospital Bad Zwischenahn; after further stations as a troop and flight physician in Leer/East Frisia and Koblenz, she served as a resident at the Federal Armed Forces Hospitals Koblenz and Ulm, Germany since 2012. Board certified in Anesthesiology since 2015. Since January 2021 senior physician at the Department of Anaesthesiology, Intensive Medicine, Emergency Medicine and Pain Therapy at the Federal Armed Forces Hospital Ulm (additional qualifications in Emergency Medicine and Special Intensive Care Medicine); numerous overseas deployments from 2009 to 2020, e.g. in Afghanistan, Mali and northern Iraq.

Dr. med. Petra Tietze-Schnur completed a degree in human medicine in Hannover, Germany, then specialist training as an anaesthetist and emergency physician in Bremen. Since 1997, she has worked in ground and air-based emergency medical services in northern Germany. Since 1997, she has been a practising Anesthesiologist in Bremerhaven, Germany. Since 2009, she has been a member of the Board of Directors of the Association for Outpatient Surgery.

Dr. med. Sven Wolf is board certified in Surgery, Orthopaedics and Trauma Surgery, Emergency Medicine and specialised Trauma Surgery. Prior to attending Medical School, he trained as a paramedic. He was senior physician in the Accident and Emergency Department at the Diakoniekrankenhaus Friederikenstift in Hannover, Germany and is now Chairman of the Department of Emergency Medicine at the DIAKOVERE Friedrikenstift and Henriettenstift in Hannover. Since 2004, he has been leading Emergency Physician of the Region/City of Hannover, Germany.

Forearm Fracture in Afghanistan 1

Björn Hossfeld

▶ There are several topics in all areas of modern medicine which have "always been done" and that are sometimes questionable in their sense—especially in the middle of the night. Quickly forgets that our modern, western medical care is still far from self-evident everywhere in the world and we should ultimately be grateful for the ubiquitous medical care. The present case shows that the conditions for many people can be quite different, or much worse.

"It's annoying!"—The clock shows 3:17 h and your eyes have just fallen shut a few minutes ago, after you as the on-call anesthesiologist had been busy for more than 11 h in the OR for countless patients. Now the surgical colleague, from the sound of his voice assumingly no less tired to conclude no less tired than yourself, is on the phone to explain that he urgently needs to make a fasciotomy to avoid a compartment syndrome in the patient with the forearm fracture already operated hours before. The question of why this is now necessary, is answered lapidar that the surgical chief physician wants it that way and—even worse—that one would have always done so.

If we are honest, there are things in all areas that "have always been done": In anesthesia, we teach the young colleagues to look into the patient's eyes during anesthesia recovery, even though the pupils dilated by excitement are practically no longer visible thanks to modern drugs. Similarly, we all learn in Medical School that a circular plaster must be split longitudinally around a fresh fracture to minimize the risk of a compartment syndrome caused by swelling.

B. Hossfeld (✉)
Department of Anesthesiology, Intensive Care, Emergency Medicine and Pain Therapy, Federal Armed Forces Hospital Ulm, Ulm, Germany
e-mail: bjoern.hossfeld@uni-ulm.de

V. Wenzel (ed.), *Case Studies in Emergency Medicine*,
https://doi.org/10.1007/978-3-662-67249-5_1

During the deployments in Afghanistan, the field hospitals of the German Armed Forces have also treated civilian local patients as part of their free capacities. In order to be treated by the NATO physicians, the patients and their relatives often undertook arduous journeys lasting several days. I remember Chafla, a small patient in the particularly cold winter of 2008. Despite the considerable snowfall and the high avalanche danger, her father set out to bring his little daughter three days long on his shoulders over difficult paths to our camp in Feyzabad. Via our interpreter we learn that the child had broken her right forearm about 10 or 12 days ago in a fall and had been treated by a local healer with a circular splint. In the following days, the little girl had complained of terrible pain, but the family had explained this with the broken bone. Then the pain had subsided, but the girl had become increasingly ill and had developed a high fever. The little patient is drowsy and tachycardic. Already during the inspection we notice the livid to black discolored fingers that protrude from the distal end of the circular bandage. The removal of this bandage reveals the full extent of the tragedy: The arm is necrotic up to the elbow, the child was clinically and proven by the laboratory results highly septic.

It is quickly clear that a timely amputation of the arm is the only option for saving our little patient. The father is informed via the interpreter and is surprisingly composed. This is an experience that we often make in this country: for the population, fatal or disfiguring diagnoses are obviously more widespread than in our Western world with medical care at the highest level available at any time of day and night and the self-image and claim to healing of our patients that has developed from this. The procedure goes smoothly and after a few days Chafla can be transferred to the Feyzabad hospital in good general condition and with unobjectionable wound conditions for further treatment, where she is still introduced to the German physicians during their joint visits with the Afghan colleagues.

Discussion

The forearm fracture is the most common bone fracture in children. In general, means the repositioning of closed fractures and subsequent immobilization, ideally in a plaster, is the correct procedure. Compartment syndrome in children is an expression of a rare (approx. 1%) multi-factorial tissue pressure increase, which is observed at the extremities, especially after trauma [1]. This can lead to compression of nerves and vessels in the affected muscle location with subsequent muscle contractures and neurological damage caused by muscle atrophy. In a well-structured medical environment with regular controls and reliable timely re-appointment of the patient with complaints, a circular plaster today offers no disadvantage compared to a primarily longitudinal split plaster [2]. It is important to recognize and correctly evaluate warning signs of complications such as pain that is barely controllable by analgesics, paresthesias and venous congestion in a timely manner. In particular, in children, the clinical signs can be unspecific or difficult to communicate; the most reliable signs of an evolving compartment syndrome were pain and increasing swelling of the extremity in one study [3]. The conservative treatment then includes above all the early splitting of constricting bandages. If the compartment syndrome is already pronounced, an emergency fasciotomy is required, the outcome is usually very good in children.

If these measures are not observed by the treating physician, this can lead to irreversible damage, as described in this case report, up to pulselessness with ischemia and necrosis. In the already septic state in which the child we treated was presented, amputation was the only causal treatment option.

1.1 Conclusion

Whenever a surgeon asks me for anaesthesia to perform a fasciotomy at night, I always remember Chafla. With her story in mind, I am always happy to get up, convinced that we can avoid the pictures our ancestors still knew.

References

1. Neiman R, Maiocco B, Deeney VF (1998) Ulnar nerve injury after closed forearm fractures in children. J Pediatr Ortho 18:683–685
2. Schulte D, Habernig S, Zuzak T, Staubli G, Altermatt S, Horst M, Garcia D (2014) Forearm fractures in children: split opinions about splitting the cast. Europ J Ped Surg 24:163–167
3. Seifert J, Matthes G, Stengel D, Hinz P, Ekkernkamp A (2002) Kompartmentsyndrom – Standards in Diagnostik und Therapie. Trauma Berufskrankh 4:101–106

24-Year-Old in a River

Sven Wolf

> Warmth, warmth, more warmth!
> For we are dying of cold
> and not darkness.
> It's not the night that kills,
> but the frost.
> de Unamuno 1972 [8]

▶ Accidental hypothermia is generally most commonly associated with accidents in connection with bodies of water, ice, snow and severe trauma. However, the classic "accidentally hypothermic, non-multiple trauma patient" in Central Europe usually only had direct contact with water or snow in about 30% of cases. About 45% of cases even occur in the "warm months" of April to September. The following example shows which aspects need to be considered in emergency medicine in the specific case.

On a cold November evening, ambulance, physician-manned ambulance and the fire department's diving team are called to a large river. In the middle of the river, which is about 100 m / 330 feet wide at this point, a 24-year-old man is swimming and calling for help. The outside temperature is 4 °C (39 °F), the water temperature is about 6 °C (43 °F). The circumstances, whether a crime or an accident, could later not be determined. In accordance with their service regulations, the fully equipped divers do not go into the water without their accompanying boat. However, this has to be carried with all participants over the stony riverbank in a time-consuming procedure. In the meantime, a policeman swims from the other riverbank to the victim. Only 17 min after arrival at the scene, both swimmers

S. Wolf (✉)
Department of Emergency Medicine, DIAKOVERE Friederikenstift, Hannover, Germany

V. Wenzel (ed.), *Case Studies in Emergency Medicine*,
https://doi.org/10.1007/978-3-662-67249-5_2

can be pulled into the inflatable boat. At hospital admission, the policeman shows signs of mild hypothermia (34.8 °C (94.6 °F) rectally) and can be discharged after outpatient warming. Somewhat somnolent, but still oriented in space and time, the 24-year-old is taken to the ambulance. Blood pressure 95/-, pulse 64. ECG: sinus rhythm with widened QRS complexes. No known comorbidities, injuries or intoxications. The target hospital now offers a possibility of maximal care 2 km / 1,2 miles away and a hospital of specialized care with cardiac surgery being 8 km / 5 miles away. The emergency physician chooses the nearby hospital. Due to the "centralized venous conditions" and the "short distance", no venous access is established. After removing the ECG cables, the young patient is transferred to the hospital by "packing, 4 men/4 corners" and moving him into the prepared intensive care bed. Immediately afterwards, he becomes unconscious and the ECG shows ventricular fibrillation. Cardiopulmonary resuscitation (CPR), acidosis correction, epinehrine and various antiarrhythmics make it possible to achieve a ventricular replacement rhythm 60 min later. Passive rewarming at an initial body core temperature of 26.8 °C (80.2 °F) (rectally) is carried out with blankets and heated infusion solutions. This makes it possible to achieve an average increase in body temperature of 1 °C (34 °F) per hour. In the following 10 h, there are recurrent episodes of ventricular fibrillation with CPR and the need to inject antiarrhythmics and to attach an external pacemaker. In the end, when ventricular fibrillation was refractory, therapy was stopped at a body core temperature of 36.9 °C (98.4 °F). Medico-legal investigation attributed the fatal outcome to resuscitation damage as an indirect accident consequence of extreme hypothermia.

Discussion
Accidental hypothermia is defined as an unwanted lowering of the core body temperature (CBT) to below 35 °C (95 °F). The staging system has now been largely standardized internationally:

- mild 35–32 °C (95–89.6 °F),
- moderate 32–28 °C (89.6–82.4 °F),
- severe/extreme: <28 °C (82.4 °F).

Accidental hypothermia is generally most often associated with accidents involving water, ice, snow and severe trauma. However, the classic "accidentally hypothermic, non-multiple trauma patient" in Central Europe usually had direct contact with water or snow in only about 30% of cases and is usually referred to as an "urban" hypothermia. About 45% of cases occur in the "warm months" of April to September. In approximately 70% of cases in Germany, the initial disease is alcohol/drug abuse or a psychiatric underlying disease [10].

While uninjured patients usually tolerate mild core body temperatures well and can be rewarmed relatively complication-free, there is a significant increase in post-traumatic complications in multiple trauma patients at a core body temperature <34 °C (<93.2 °F), primarily coagulopathy [1].

The incidence of accidental hypothermia in multiple trauma is given as 12 to 66%, the increased mortality in the coincidence of both is between 30 and 80% [3, 5].

With decreasing core body temperature, stage-related tables with pathophysiological changes, such as somnolence and unconsciousness, can be found in textbooks. However, in pre-hospital emergency medical service practice, the clinical parameters of the inhomogeneous patient population rarely correspond to the textbook tables. So foot-walking 29.2 °C (84.6 °F) cold patients are just as likely to be found as completely conscious, subjectively symptom-free homeless people with a core body temperature of 26.7 °C (80.1 °F) [9]. In addition to influences on vigilance, reduced metabolism rates/cytoprotective effects, reversible thrombocyte/thrombin and fibrin function disorders, electrolyte shifts and changes in myocardial membrane potentials are observed with resulting rigidity, increased irritability and high risk of life-threatening rhythm disorders (especially ventricular fibrillation) by mechanical and thermal triggers. The latter also pathophysiologically prepares the ground for the so-called "rescue death" [1, 9]. Even in clinical suspicion of moderate or severe/extreme accidental hypothermia, rough manipulations of the patient by turning over, lifting from the horizontal or even the position for rectal temperature measurement must be avoided. Both directly by the manipulation and indirectly by the backflow of cold "shell blood" from the periphery to central, in addition to a further drop in core body temperature, the increased cardiac irritability can lead to malignant arrhythmias/ventricular fibrillation as mechanical and thermal triggers. Swimming, severely or extremely cooled patients are also subject to another pathophysiology of the "rescue death": With centralized circulation and reduced cardiac function, the hydrostatic pressure of the surrounding water can be the decisive factor for a just sufficient cardiac output. A sudden rescue from the supportive hydrostatic pressure conditions in combination with an increase in orthostatic pressure during vertical rescue (e.g. hoisting by an EMS helicopter) and an increased demand on cardiac output can lead to a decisive reduction in coronary perfusion with heart failure [2, 4]. Further, with accidental hypothermia associated terms such as "afterdrop" and "rewarming shock" are phenomena of clinical therapy and should not be discussed here.

In particular, in the case of drowning accidents in cold water, the tolerance to hypoxia is increased by hypothermia. Duration and speed of cooling are among the decisive factors for the outcome. The lowest recorded accidental hypothermia is 13.7 °C (56.7 °F) [1]; successful passive rewarming from extreme hypothermia with continuous CPR for more than 4 h with uneventful neurological outcome has also been described [6, 7]! The well-known saying results from such case reports:

Nobody is dead until rewarmed and dead.

It should be mentioned at this point that confirmed submersion or hypoxia times of significantly more than 60 min also have no chance of a complete recovery in extreme hypothermia. Tympanic thermometers/ear infrared thermometers are already available more often for temperature measurement on site. Even if they do not exactly correspond to the esophageal and deep rectal measurement, for example in the case of water in the ear canal, they can confirm the suspicion of accidental hypothermia. If only a conventional stick thermometer is available and if the external circumstances ("Environment") alone justify the mere suspicion of a significant hypothermia, rectal measurements on site must be omitted and the patient must be hospitalized as quickly as possible with the provisional diagnosis "severe hypothermia".

A significant decision for the later outcome of the severely/extremely hypothermic patient is made by the emergency physician on site with the choice of the target hospital [1, 9]. Sufficient rewarming is hardly possible and promising prehospitally, except on board of larger rescue cruisers. The priority is to maintain heat with blankets, ambulance heating, warmed infusion solutions and, for example, in traffic accidents with 1000-watt spotlights from the fire brigade. In the hospital/intensive care unit, rewarming rates of 1 °C (34 °F)/hour are generally possible with all conceivable external methods, even during resuscitation [9]. However, during resuscitation conditions, a significantly increased personnel requirement is inevitably unavoidable. With an extracorporeal circulation on a heart-lung machine, warming rates >11 °C (52 °F)/h are possible.

2.1   Conclusion

The prehospital diagnosis of "accidental hypothermia" can sometimes be significantly hampered if the external circumstances do not immediately draw the attention of the emergency physician. A complication-free diagnostic certainty is offered here by the commercially available ear infrared thermometer. In case of suspicion of moderate or severe hypothermia, all gross manipulations and repositioning of the patient must be avoided. Once the indication for CPR is given, it must be consistently and comprehensively continued throughout transport. An important decision for the outcome is already made on site with the selection of the target hospital and the potential possibility of extracorporeal circulation/heart-lung machine.

References

1. Andruszkow H, Hildebrand F (2014) Akzidentelle Hypothermie/schwere Unterkühlung. Notarzt 30:7–15
2. Golden FS (1982) Der heutige Stand der Unterkühlungsbehandlung. In: Unterkühlung im Seenotfall – 2. Symposium 1982 in Cuxhaven der DGzRS, Symposiumsband, DGzRS Bremen
3. Gregory JS, Flancbaum L, Townsend, et al (1991) Incidence and timing of hypothermia in trauma patients undergoing operations. J Trauma 31:1247–1252
4. Hauty MG, Esrig BC, Hill JG, Long WB (1987) Prognostic factors in severe accidental hypothermia: the hood tragedy. J Trauma 27:1107–1112
5. Hildebrand F, Probst C, Frink M, Huber-Wagner S, Krettek C (2009) Bedeutung der Hypothermie beim Polytrauma. Unfallchirurg 112:959–964
6. Lexow K (1991) Severe accidental hypothermia: survival after 6 hours 30 minutes of cardiopulmonary resuscitation. Arctic Med Res 50(Suppl 6):112–114
7. Roggero E, Stricker H, Biegger P (1992) Akzidentelle Hypothermie mit kardiopulmonalen Stellstand: prolongierte Reanimation ohne extrakorporellen Kreislauf. Schweiz Med Wochenschr 1:161–164
8. de Unamuno M (1972) The tragic sense of life in men and in nations. Princeton University Press, Princeton
9. Wolf S (1996) Akzidentelle Hypothermie in Norddeutschland (1983–1993) – Eine therapeutische Herausforderung -. Inaugural-Dissertation Georg-August-Universität Göttingen
10. Wolf S (2000) Kältetod – Wie oft schlägt er wirklich zu? Inzidenz, Mortalität und Morbidität der Hypothermie. In: Turner E, Kaudasch G (Hrsg) Unterkühlung im Rettungsdienst – Prä- und innerklinische Therapie der akzidentelle Hypothermie. Pabst Science Publ., Lengerich.

Serious Traffic Accident in Fog

Martin Messelken

▶ In emergency medicine, one often encounters situations that do not develop as expected and therefore require improvisational skills. The good or bad environmental conditions also play a corresponding role. In the present case, the situation of a triage at the accident site after a traffic accident is presented, as well as some possible difficulties that may arise in this constellation for the deployment team.

A car occupied by a young family has an accident on a foggy Sunday morning in the early 1980s. The accident site is at the outer edge of the rural EMS service area; therefore, a travel time of 17 min for the ambulance and EMS is not unusual. Based on the accident report, the EMS dispatch center sends the only available physician-manned ambulance and two ambulances. The following scene presents itself to the arriving EMS workers: The car had overturned in a long left-hand bend and was back on its wheels on a sloping meadow. The driver (mother) is slightly dazed but apparently physically largely unharmed; the probably intoxicated passenger (father), on the other hand, is hanging lifelessly in the safety belt. He has vomited and his cervical spine appears unstable. Given the fact that two unconscious children, aged 4 and 6, are lying motionless on the back seats, any cardiopulmonary resuscitation attempt of the man is omitted. After this triage and the prospect of not being able to receive any support from a helicopter EMS (fog) or a nearby physician (busy with different emergency case) at the moment, the children are brought individually into the ambulance and treated one after the other by the doctor. The older of the two girls has a clear pupil difference with a Glasgow Coma Scale (GCS) of 6, she is first given analgesia and then intubated. The manual ventilation is handed over to an experienced paramedic. After the

M. Messelken (✉)
Bad Boll, Germany
e-mail: m.messelken@gmail.com

V. Wenzel (ed.), *Case Studies in Emergency Medicine*,
https://doi.org/10.1007/978-3-662-67249-5_3

second girl (also Glasgow Coma Scale of 6) has been given analgesia and intubated, both endotracheal tubes have been clinically and auscultatorily verified and fixed in their correct position, the monitoring of the circulatory system in both children does not give any indication of further injuries or a volume deficit. In the responsible hospital for maximum care, two ventilated children with isolated head and brain trauma are then registered; the transport takes place in a convoy. During the transport, the physician constantly informs himself by radio contact regarding the situation in the other ambulance; a stop is made for visual inspection of the findings in between. The mother arrives at the hospital in a police car, where she is given pastoral care.

The trauma surgery hospital has gathered the usual personnel available on a Sunday morning, as well as the on-call staff of the anesthesia and children's hospital, in the emergency room; the handover takes place about 70 min after the accident. The radiological diagnosis in the 6-year-old girl with manifest anisocoria shows the finding of a subdural bleed, which results in a craniotomy carried out quickly. However, despite maximum therapy, the death within the first 24 h as a result of the brain injuries could not be averted. The 4-year-old sister has a clear contusion with brain edema; after adequate intensive care treatment, she can be discharged 6 weeks later without any residuals and today lives with her own family.

Discussion

Triage at the scene of an accident (i.e. sorting and classifying the medical assistance needed) has the highest priority in the event of a fully occupied car. Due to the unfavorable existing structures (weekday = Sunday, weather = fog, personnel and vehicle availability = severe restrictions), there was already a significant imbalance of personnel and material from the outset, which could not be improved in the course of the event. Therefore, the care provided by the only emergency physician and the ambulance teams focused on the seriously injured children; all other decisions, such as driving to a single destination hospital, are due to this fact. From today's perspective, two ground-based emergency medical systems and one EMS helicopter would be the appropriate staffing to establish a 1:1 care situation. In the absence of suitable transport ventilators and ventilation monitoring, ventilation was carried out manually and without accompanying capnometry. The possible and to be assumed hyperventilation condition could not only be disadvantageous in this case—a mild hyperventilation during controlled conditions is to be aimed for in the initial treatment of a patient with craniocerebral trauma. The distribution of patients to several hospitals or a trauma center would have been the next logical step. The fact that two seriously injured children had to be admitted to one hospital—and on a Sunday morning—is unfavorable and only justified by the fact that a convoy had to be transported without delay. Today, however, a strategy of spatial dislocation would be clearly favored. When I was the first arriving EMS helicopter physician [1] years later, this question did not arise at all; there were sufficient ground-based emergency physicians available within the specified time frame, so that the patients, including two children with severe head trauma, could be transported to different hospitals with EMS accompaniment.

3.1 Conclusion

There will always be situations in EMS that require a considerable amount of improvisation. Good structural quality and trained processes that can be oriented to established algorithms are very helpful in actually implementing a "Plan B". Early communication with the medical facilities to which you transport seriously injured patients is also very important.

References

1. Gries A et al (2008) Time in care of trauma patients in the air rescue service: implications for disposition? Anaesthesist 57(6):562–570

80-Year-Old Patient with Devastating Chest Pain

Luise Schnitzer

▶ This case very clearly shows that it is not always easy to put the symptoms present together at the place of use to form a coherent picture and that it must not be underestimated how often a selective perception makes the past medical history more difficult, in the sense of: "What may not be, that can not be!"

We are alarmed at 2:47 pm with the message "severe chest pain" and set out to treat a "routine case". We are received by the patient's husband, who introduces himself as a retired physician and leads us to his wife, who is lying on the sofa, groaning quietly and very pale. The patient only reacts with the groaning already heard. I try to quickly assess the circulation parameters and have to conclude that no pulse is palpable. As a result, I arrange for our patient to be placed on the floor so that a good starting position for an effective resuscitation attempt is created. The woman reacts to these measures with groaning: we raise the legs to improve the circulation first. Meanwhile, I try to get information about the starting situation, to access the patient and to write an ECG. The technical processes run smoothly, but the past medical history is difficult.

According to the husband, the 80-year-old patient has always been healthy and does not take any medication. The evening before, she had felt a little weak for the first time and had once vomited blood. After that she had felt better again. She had not complained of any pain and therefore the couple had gone to bed. It may be surprising that the retired physician husband underestimated the situation to such an extent, but sometimes the desire and the will are stronger than the mind: "What may not be, that can not be". "His wife had always been healthy and mobile, had

L. Schnitzer (✉)
Charité University Medicine Berlin, Campus Benjamin Franklin, Department of Cardiology and Pulmology, Berlin, Germany

© The Author(s), under exclusive license to Springer-Verlag GmbH, DE, part of Springer Nature 2023
V. Wenzel (ed.), *Case Studies in Emergency Medicine*,
https://doi.org/10.1007/978-3-662-67249-5_4

taken care of him and supported him in everything—and now it is simply impossible that she could be sick and can no longer do it!"

During the day she had felt a little weak and therefore he had suggested to her to get some fresh air. They had also set out for a walk, but his wife had fainted after a short distance, had vomited or coughed up blood again, so they had broken off the walk and started the way home. On the last stage, however, he had to "pull" his wife almost home. I only receive these details with difficulty because the helpless husband does not fully understand the situation and keeps asking his wife for confirmation, which she can not give him because of her condition.

In the meantime, the ECG was written: unremarkable finding, no end-point changes, no rhythm disorders and no evidence of ischemia. However, the patient is relatively bradycardic with a heart rate of 57/min, the blood pressure is now measurable at 50 mmHg systolic, the oxygen saturation cannot be detected at the low blood pressure. Overall, the review of the circulatory situation does not reveal any significant change, so that, based on the previous history and the patient's pallor, a severe gastrointestinal bleed moves to the forefront of the differential diagnoses, especially since the patient is now vomiting fresh blood again. A second, large-lumen intravenous catheter is inserted and infusions are running through both intravenous lines. An inspection of the skin does not reveal any evidence of liver disease, such as spider naevi or increased and thickened veins on the abdomen in the sense of a caput medusae; the liver is palpable at the costal margin, not hard or enlarged. Questions to the husband do not reveal any evidence of past hepatitis or increased alcohol consumption. My thoughts are interrupted by an increasing bradycardia and then an asystole, so that I now put the patient into anesthesia, have chest compressions performed and intubated, and to my surprise have to find that fresh blood has to be suctioned out of the trachea as well.

After injection of 2 mg of epinephrine in total, the heart rhythm remains stable, the blood pressure also rises again to 50 mmHg through the infusion of 2000 ml of crystalloid solution, and I arrange for the transport to the hospital. I am aware that I cannot achieve any significant improvement here on site and that a diagnosis is urgently required to find the source of the bleed—it just doesn't become clear where the blood loss is coming from. A bleed from an ulcer ventriculior duodeni is quite possible, but the course seems too fulminant to me. With an oesophageal varices bleed I would have expected a correspondingly larger visible blood loss. The bleed from the trachea completely confuses me—this seems to be more in total than the vomited blood. Fresh blood has to be suctioned off again and again.

A pulmonary bleed, such as from vessel erosion in bronchial cancer, can be significant and could explain the patient's overall condition. However, the past medical history does not suggest a pulmonary condition—neither cough nor exertional dyspnea. Within 10 min—at 3:35 PM—we reach the hospital, and, due to my pre-registration—"unclear severe bleed with unstable circulation—possibly pulmonary or gastrointestinal," everything is prepared. A blood gas analysis shows a hemoglobin level of 8.5 g/dl, the pH is 6.96, pCO_2 46 mmHg, pO_2 249 mmHg—after 1 h 105 mmHg. The chest X-ray shows a heart of normal size, the mediastinum is not widened, no effusion or infiltrate, but a finding left basal, which is compatible with an aspiration pneumonia.

In the CT of the chest, there are several penetrating ulcerations in the distal part of the atherosclerotic-changed descending aorta over a length of approximately 5 cm at the level of thoracic vertebrae 10/11. In addition, an accompanying intramural hematoma and a questionable covered perforation to the left lateral lobe are shown, no pleural effusion and no ascites. As on the chest X-ray, an aspiration is shown in the left lower lobe. Due to the questionable covered perforation to the left lateral lobe, the patient is taken to interventional radiology without further delay and treated with a thoracic stent; in rehabilitation treatment, the patient ultimately recovers completely without further complications and is discharged home.

Discussion

This case has remained particularly memorable to me because I found it so difficult to interpret the findings and to put them into an understandable context. A cardiac cause was unlikely due to the ECG findings, and the findings of coughing up and vomiting blood spoke against an aortic dissection. The amount of blood that was visible did not fit with the circulatory collapse, nor did the bradycardia, which rather pointed to a cardiac event than to massive bleeding. An aortic aneurysm with fistula formation in the esophagus or trachea is a very rare complication and is associated with a high mortality rate [1]. The literature reports an incidence of 0.35–1.6%—and in most cases it is a late complication of an aneurysm operation [2, 3]. Many patients with a thoracic aortic aneurysm initially have completely non-specific symptoms and are often treated for completely different diseases, such as back pain or upper gastrointestinal bleeding, without evidence of a bleeding source. The symptoms are also difficult to interpret because the pain can radiate to very different body regions and can be bilateral, so that the diagnosis, as in this case, can only be made by the acute deterioration. Here the question arises quickly how the patient is to be treated—does the thoracic aortic aneurysm have to be operated on by cardiac or vascular surgeons or is an endovascular treatment possible in interventional radiology [3, 4]?

A small side issue in this case may also be the dramatic underestimation of his wife's illness by her husband, the physician. How is it possible to overlook such signs? It must not be underestimated that a selective perception often makes the past medical history more difficult—which colleague has not already experienced that, despite a thorough and comprehensive anamnesis, the decisive hint is only mentioned in a banal aside or—even worse—during the chief physician's round. Certainly the case would have been better and less dramatic to treat if the husband had presented his wife to the hospital the evening before. However, this question can only be answered speculatively—a bleeding source would probably not have been found by gastroenterologists. A CT or MRI scan would probably have detected the ulcerating plaques, but the question remains whether an indication for surgery would have been made.

4.1 Conclusion

A thoracic aortic aneurysm can cause a variety of non-specific symptoms, but can then lead to extremely rapid blood pressure drops in the event of (covered) rupture. In this case it was important to drive quickly to the hospital in the unclear situation in order to initiate a targeted therapy quickly.

References

1. Kokatnur L, Rudrappa M (2015) Primary aorto-esophageal fistula: Great masquerader of esophageal variceal bleeding. Indian J Crit Care Med 19(2):119–121
2. Chiba D, Hanabata N, Araki Y, Sawaya M, Yoshimura T, Aoki M, Shimoyama T, Fukuda S (2013) Aortoesophageal fistula after thoracic endovascular aortic repair diagnosed and followed with endoscopy. Intern Med 52(4):451–455
3. Hyhlik-Dürr A, Geisbüsch R, Hakimi M, Weber TF, Schaible A, Böckler B (2009) Endovaskuläre Aortenchirurgie: Management sekundärer aortobronchialer – und enteraler Fisteln. Chirurg 80:947–955
4. Chad Hughes G (2015) Management od acute type B aortic dissektion: ADSORB trial. J Thorac Cardiovasc Surg 149(2 Suppl):S158–S162

Joachim Koppenberg

▶ In the present case it becomes clear that one has to accept in some exceptional cases that the patient's situation deteriorates initially through the measures taken, but this may be unavoidable in order to save him. And sometimes a second attempt is necessary to achieve the desired goal.

As a motivated junior resident in anesthesia and with 2 years of experience as an emergency physician in ground-based emergency services, I had a previously quiet ambulance service on a Monday after a free weekend—including a hearty breakfast and the latest "gossip" from the weekend with the on-duty paramedics. Around 10:00 clock the EMS control center alarms us to an "unconscious person" in a forwarding company. Since the forwarding company is located a little outside the city in an industrial area and we are on the way in a compact physician-manned ambulance from the university hospital, the EMS control center alarms an ambulance stationed about 6 min from the scene of the accident in parallel. So the journey continues to be relaxed: A vanguard is on the way, so there will be twice as many paramedics at the scene of the emergency as usual, and in the case of unconsciousness it is probably once again one of the numerous urban hypoglycemias or epileptic seizures that would be awake again when we arrived. So: "Everything is relaxed"! My relaxation is quickly gone after our arrival 14 min later. The ambulance crew arrived a few minutes before us and presented an initially very confusing situation: An approximately 40-year-old worker is lying with severe, bleeding facial injuries on his back a few meters from a truck. Near the loading area is a large pool of blood, a blood trail leads from there to the lying

J. Koppenberg (✉)
Department of Anesthesiology, Pain Therapy and Emergency Medicine, OSPIDAL – Center da sandà Engiadina Bassa, Scuol, Switzerland
e-mail: Joachim.Koppenberg@cseb.ch

© The Author(s), under exclusive license to Springer-Verlag GmbH, DE, part of Springer Nature 2023
V. Wenzel (ed.), *Case Studies in Emergency Medicine*,
https://doi.org/10.1007/978-3-662-67249-5_5

patient. There are no further clues to the accident at this time, as the only witness to the accident is under severe "shock" (here the unfortunate term of shock is meant as it is described in the newspaper). Several employees of the forwarding company are running around excitedly. The ambulance crew has already attached an ECG (heart rate 44/min) and taken a blood pressure measurement (systolic 80 mmHg, diastolic unmeasurable), the oxygen saturation is 66%. During the first orienting examination, a Glasgow Coma Scale (GCS) of 3, a shattered lower jaw, multiple fractures of the middle face and blood loss from both ear canals are found. Further injuries cannot be ascertained in the short time available. The nose-throat-space is completely filled with blood and more and more blood is gushing out of the mouth. Respiratory mechanics can only be determined to a limited extent. Due to the existing findings, it is quickly clear that the patient needs an airway securing as soon as possible, independent of the accident mechanism or other injuries and further differentiated treatment measures, since the pronounced hypoxia already induces bradycardia and announces an impending cardiac arrest. Due to the shattered lower jaw and the severe bleeding, the Swiss army knife and the ballpoint pen for the emergency cricothyroidotomy are going through my head—I had never performed this measure before, except on a dead sheep. Fortunately, one of the older paramedics hands me the laryngoscope and a tube and says calmly: "Try it—I'll get the cricothyroidotomy set from the ambulance while I'm at it." Before starting an IV or administering any drugs with a Glasgow Coma Scale of 3, the oral intubation is surprisingly easy and problem-free, with simultaneous suctioning. In the case of a suspected fall from the back of a truck, we carry out intubation while manually stabilizing the neck. While the intubation is being carried out, a paramedic is able to successfully insert a 16-gauge needle into the left forearm. Despite the overall more difficult personnel management (four paramedics are working from two sets of equipment and there are several excited workers around the treatment area), after the airway is secured with an unexpectedly easy intubation and the IV is in place, I slowly start to feel again: "We've got this under control!" After checking the correct endotracheal tube placement with capnography, the difficult tube fixation due to the heavy bleeding in the face, and the application of a neck brace, a large amount of blood can be suctioned through the tube. After ventilation with 100% oxygen, the peripheral oxygen saturation rises to 94% and, as a result, the heart rate gradually increases to 122/min (physiology should be right again), while the blood pressure remains systolic at 80 mmHg. With the working diagnosis of "severe head injury", it is clear that we need to aggressively treat hypotension in order to maintain cerebral perfusion pressure (cerebral perfusion pressure = mean arterial pressure minus intracranial pressure) and get to the hospital as quickly as possible (the principle of "load and play"). The already inserted IV access "runs well" (already 1000 ml of full electrolyte solution and 500 ml of balanced HAES solution have flowed through) and so the idea is to prepare for transport, to insert a second IV access. I feel a certain inner satisfaction—everything is going well. But before I insert the second access, the patient suddenly becomes bradycardic and shortly afterwards even asystolic. At the same time, one of the many paramedics hangs on the already inserted venous access and pulls it out unintentionally. Both happen so quickly that I am speechless and helpless for a short time. However, I quickly have to admit that this is probably not a good time to rethink my career choice. The only good news: The bleeding has stopped! After I have accepted the new situation internally and the paramedics have already started chest compressions, I motivate myself with the fact that it is at least an observed cardiac arrest from the perspective of cardiac arrest and the patient is already intubated. So we only need a new IV access to fulfill the "duty" resuscitation, which is quickly done. The initiated cardiopulmonary resuscitation runs smoothly and in accordance with the guideline Asystole—there are also enough rescuers on site. After the mandatory part of the resuscitation runs well, we come to the elective: Why did the patient have a cardiac arrest? So we go through the classic H's and T's of the potentially reversible causes:

- Hypoxia?—The patient is well oxygenated, the tube is still in the right place.
- Hypovolemia?—With the bleeding in principle possible, but we treat it already aggressively.
- Hypothermia? This is extremely unlikely due to the sudden accident and so slowly we were not at the scene of the accident.
- Hypo-, hyperkalemia, hypokalemia? This is also unlikely as the trigger of the accident in a 40-year-old worker.
- Pericardial tamponade? In principle possible, but the leading injury is in the head/neck area.
- Intoxication? There are no indications for this.
- Thromboembolism? Also very unlikely due to the accident.
- Tension pneumothorax?—There are no obvious injury indications for this, but we do not know the accident mechanism yet.

On re-auscultation, there is a significantly weakened left breathing sound compared to the auscultation after intubation, and it seems that the ventilation pressure is increasing on the ventilator bag. So the working hypothesis is tension pneumothorax, and I puncture in the sense of a (test) or relief puncture with a 14-G needle in the second intercostal space medioclavicular left (Monaldi)—promptly and pleasingly there is the expected hissing escape of air. But unfortunately, the target size of a relief puncture is not "hissing escape of air", but the improvement of the cardiovascular situation, which does not occur. The patient remains asystolic and resuscitation-worthy. After this new disappointment, resignation now sets in for everyone—we unsuccessfully resuscitate a 40-year-old multiple trauma patient and begin to discuss the meaning of our efforts or the termination of the measures. After a short pause, I decide to give the patient a proper thoracic drainage by means of a blunt minithoracotomy in the front axillary line in the 4./5. Intercostal space (chest tube) and, if the situation remains unchanged, to discontinue the resuscitation attempt. After piercing the pleura with the index finger, there is again a hissing escape of air—but now, contrary to my expectation, a prompt transition to a sinus rhythm (heart rate 90/min) with ejection and a blood pressure of 60 mmHg systolic. Now we transport the patient to the hospital as quickly as possible and try to stabilize systolic blood pressure as well as possible with volume and catecholamines during the journey; diastolic, however, no blood pressure is measurable anymore. In the hospital, the patient is quickly massively transfused, tracheotomized and operated upon—but unfortunately dies shortly afterwards from the consequences of the severe head injury.

Discussion

This intervention taught me some important things that I could only really understand after several conversations and literature research, but which have had a lasting effect on my understanding and approach to severely injured patients. First, the question arose as to why the patient could develop a tension pneumothorax so quickly, which even caused a cardiac arrest. As it turned out later, when unloading the truck, a so-called jumbo pallet fell on the patient's head/chest area, which was immediately lifted away by a forklift driver to free the patient. This is how the obviously severe head injuries and, as the autopsy showed, a single isolated rib fracture originated. There was probably also a minimal pleura injury. However, since the patient hardly or not at all breathed spontaneously due to the other injuries, no relevant tension pneumothorax could develop at first. But then we—the rescuers—intubated the patient and carried out positive pressure ventilation and—oh wonder—operated the tension valve mechanism with each ventilation stroke. So we actively triggered the tension pneumothorax, which drove the patient into cardiac arrest. The pressure generated by the ventilation creates a constantly increasing pressure in the pleural space. And why didn't the relief puncture with the 14-gauge needle produce a better result? Well, we were basically right, but again: The target size of the relief of a pneumothorax is not "hissing escape of air", but an improvement in the cardiopulmonary situation. The following reasons can explain the failure of the needle puncture method: Either the pleura closed the plastic cannula again or it bent it over or there was a hemopneumothorax and we only relieved a small, nonrelevant part of the pneumothorax [2–4]. However, the decisive finding is that in the event of an unsuccessful needle relief puncture, a "proper" thoracic drainage must always and consistently be placed, as a needle puncture can not be sufficient. Especially in the resuscitation situation, the S-3 guideline multiple trauma therefore recommends the consistent exclusion of a tension pneumothorax as the cause of cardiac arrest by possibly also placing a thoracic drainage on both sides [1].

5.1   Conclusion

The switch from spontaneous to mechanical ventilation after intubation can trigger a tension pneumothorax! This means in concrete terms: Whoever intubates a patient with thoracic trauma must practically wait for the tension pneumothorax (circulatory depression, increase in ventilation pressure) and then treat the resulting tension pneumothorax consistently—otherwise the rescuer unintentionally triggered cardiac arrest! If there is suspicion of a tension pneumothorax, a needle-relief puncture can be carried out first. However, if this does not show the desired clinical effect, a sufficient thoracic drainage must be carried out on both sides.

References

1. Deutsche Gesellschaft für Unfallchirurgie (2022) S3- Leitlinien Polytrauma/ Schwerstverletzten-Behandlung. awmf-Register Nr. 187-023, www.awmf.org. Accessed 15 July 2023
2. Dominquez KM, Ekeh AP, Tchorz KM et al (2013) Is routine tube thoracostomy necessary after prehospital needle decompression for tension pneumothorax? Am J Surg 205(3):329–332
3. Inaba K, Branco BC, Eckstein M et al (2011) Optimal positioning for emergent needle thoracostomy: a cadaver-based study. J Trauma 51(5):1099–1110
4. Mistry N, Bleetman A, Roberts KJ (2009) Chest decompression during resuscitation of patients in prehospital traumatic cardiac arrest. Emerg Med J 16(10):738–740

The Final Exam

6

Volker Wenzel

▶ Studying human medicine, like many other courses of study, is a great challenge for the young people studying it. The present case is concerned with the fact that this challenge cannot be mastered by everyone without support and accompaniment and can become overwhelming.

A colleague told me that he had got to know a very smart medical student when he was on duty as an emergency physician who was looking for an M.D. thesis; however, he was just busy with tedious exams, so we planned to include him in a project six months later. He was then very pleased to get to know the scientific side of his studies and worked on his M.D. thesis with a huge amount of energy and personal commitment. The M.D. thesis developed excellently. He had an extremely good sense of humour—for example, he said that he would need an exit clause in a residency physician contract in case he could become a soccer coach at a well-known club. Once he asked me to postpone an appointment by one day just before he handed in his M.D. thesis because he had to help out in the EMS. The next day he came into the office with sunburn on his arms and face. In response to my ironic question as to whether work in the EMS had been very hard, he replied with disarming honesty: We were lying in a deckchair and fell asleep in the sun— whether on standby in the EMS station or in the mountains, he left charismatically open. I thought to myself: That was a white lie!, but obviously he wanted to break out once more just before the end of his time in Medical School, before the working day started. I also recognised a little of myself in this M.D. thesis student and was therefore also lenient with him: Like him, I lost my father as a child, like him,

V. Wenzel (✉)
Department of Anesthesiology, Intensive Care, Emergency Medicine, and Pain Therapy,
Friedrichshafen Regional Medical Center and Tettnang Hospital, Friedrichshafen, Germany
e-mail: v.wenzel@klinikum-fn.de

V. Wenzel (ed.), *Case Studies in Emergency Medicine*,
https://doi.org/10.1007/978-3-662-67249-5_6

I had to work a lot during my time in Medical School to finance everything. A little later the M.D. thesis was finished and I sent it to the dean's office. The next day I got a call: "We cannot process this M.D. thesis, after all, most of the course certificates are missing!" I called the M.D. thesis student and left a message on his mobile phone asking for clarification. The next day he called back and said: Everything clarified—he was confused, as was also the case with a fellow student, because the Dean's office had moved. The following day, the Dean's office called me again and they told me: "We have checked everything again, but it remains the same: Going forward is not possible at this time because most of the coursework is still missing." I was completely shocked. Every attempt to reach the M.D. thesis student failed; he also did not call back the next day. Another day later, he did not show up at his part-time job at an EMS station, which had never happened before. The research showed that he had not returned from a mountain hike as announced. The mountain rescue service was deployed and searched the mountains all night; the next morning, a helicopter flew over the area. They finally found him dead at the foot of a cliff; he had fallen about 150 m. The call about his death hit me like a lightning bolt. I was paralyzed. Every year, dozens of recreational athletes die in the Tyrolean mountains—tobogganists and skiers collide with trees, climbers lose their grip, the altitude in combination with great effort causes heart attacks, paragliders crash, kayakers drown—often bad equipment or an unfortunate assessment of the weather and the mountains was an important factor that led to the accident. But our M.D. thesis student had always been very conscientious on his mountain hikes and he was extremely experienced. All circumstances undoubtedly pointed to the fact that this was not a tragic accident, but a carefully prepared suicide. We researched that our M.D. thesis student probably wanted to gain time with a lie about successfully completed exams at the time of the aforementioned "annoying exams" in order to escape his exam anxiety. Since his descriptions of these (allegedly successful) exams were absolutely plausible, the facade worked—possibly even to his own surprise. Of course, he received messages from the Dean's office at the beginning of each semester about outstanding exams, but he paid his semester fees reliably and thus did not stand out in the system. We had not asked for a copy of his coursework in our research laboratory for his work, because he worked on his project with great joy, commitment and success—no wonder, after all, he did not have to take an exam with us, but only write an M.D. thesis—which he did brilliantly. In this way, a double life developed, which he was able to maintain due to his high intelligence and his impressive charisma. But of course the air got thinner and thinner; one year before his death, he announced the end of his studies "in two semesters". In this time he bloomed again through a variety of great leisure experiences—only one colleague noticed one week before his death that he looked very thoughtful for someone who had actually just successfully completed Medical School. But at that time our M.D. thesis student had probably already decided that there was no way back into the real world—there were dozens of opportunities when we could have helped him. Everyone in his large circle of friends and colleagues and I would have immediately dropped everything to help him. But he decided to continue his legend, which he probably considered to be irreversible at some point—he deceived to avoid disappointing his entire environment—and paid for it with his life.

Discussion
In the USA, there are very detailed studies on the suicidality of medical students [1]. In a survey at the University of Michigan in Ann Arbor, 46% of medical students said they had had depressive phases, 15% had been diagnosed with depression once, and 4% had seriously considered suicide during their medical studies [2]. Compared to earlier (approx. 1960–1980) reports from German universities with suicide rates of 35–61 per 100,000 students, the Innsbruck figures with 36 suicides per 100,000 medical students are lower, but still more than twice as high as in the age-appropriate comparison group (approx. 17 per 100,000) or in American medical students from an earlier study (16 per 100,000) [3].

Important risk factors for suicide are depression, bipolar disorder, schizophrenia, and borderline personality disorder; 90% of suicides have one of these conditions [4]. Student life away from stabilizing social structures, financial dependence despite higher age, the high pressure of work in a mass study, the predominant and one-sided "mental work", identity problems, fears of the future and of existence, and an unclear social status were also identified as important risk factors for suicidality of students. The exact reasons for a student suicide therefore appear to be diverse; a fatal combination of character traits, life circumstances, mental state and stressful events seems to be decisive. There are hardly any clear signs in the run-up to suicides as with other diseases; doctors, friends and relatives are often unsure and therefore cannot clearly assess how serious the danger actually is. People in emotional distress often lack the necessary courage to seek professional help [5].

In addition to the classical risk factors, deep narcissistic injuries with fears of social reputation loss can also be causes of suicides—especially in highly respected medicine. Our performance society favors competition and winner types, which can create a tension field between unrealistic expectations and personal performance. Overwhelming ideals of how one should be can be dictated by both external and internal factors. The higher the target state is set, the deeper the humiliating crash in the form of a final failure in the study can be.

The allocation of Medical School slots is largely based on the final grade or the Medical Aptitude Test and thus selects people who can quickly learn theoretical subject matter. Other important key qualifications such as sociability, empathy, social competence and (self-)organizational talent are thus left out of account, but are very important for the study success of a medical student and for the further professional success of a physician. In Medical School, the acceptance and coping with failure in exams may be an unexpected and drastic change for which, up to that point, the performance-oriented and success-spoiled high school graduates usually did not have to learn any coping strategies. Furthermore, a disillusionment often develops during Medical School, because the private and professional future is increasingly assessed as realistic and therefore demotivating due to high workload, moderate salary and high sacrifices in private life [6].

A way out of this dilemma of an increased suicide rate among medical students is primary prevention in order to mitigate the effect of stressors in studies within the framework of a solidary coexistence. While fellow students can assess each other's living conditions well in order to, for example, notice excessive alcohol consumption or social withdrawal, university staff are among others required to request explanations for lack of progress in studies carefully and binding. For this it is necessary to de-taboo the topic "psychological stress" in Medical School. An open approach to the topic could serve the transfer of coping strategies for stressors and remove the reluctance to seek professional help. Likewise, university staff should not only convey pure subject matter, but also with the student's life goals and tasks beyond profession and career and promote them in their personal development process or refer them to appropriate counseling centers [7]. Two years later I examined a student who submitted a confident performance in the internship, but had a complete "blackout" in the formal examination. I asked her to solve this phenomenon with professional help, because otherwise she would always be below her actual value in a pressure situation. Weeks later she reported back and told me proudly that she had solved the problem with the help of the psychological student counseling. Counseling and help is therefore possible, but one has to talk about it—one only gets help if one asks for it. The Corona pandemic has shown that personal encounters and leisure activities have been significantly restricted by the different lockdown levels, which in turn potentially unstable people further unsettled. Consequently, it has become even more difficult to assess the real well-being of another person.

6.1 Conclusion

Our M.D. thesis student's case shows that trust in people is good, but a check is required to confirm the trust—whether a check of the course certificates would have saved this life, however, is unclear. The suicide risk of medical students compared to the general population appears to be increased, but we do not know whether our observations can be transferred to other universities because of missing comparative data. Apparently, it is not a single specific event that moves medical students to suicide, but a combination of individual risk factors and the social environment. Unfortunately, this problem is currently not receiving the necessary attention. The Corona pandemic has made digital meetings much better and available, so that better help can be given—if it is also used.

References

1. Dyrbye LN, Thomas MR, Massie FS, Power DV, Eacker A, Harper W, Durning S, Moutier C, Szydlo DW, Novotny PJ, Sloan JA, Shanafelt TD (2008) Burnout and suicidal ideation among US medical students. Ann Intern Med 149:334–341
2. Schwenk TL, Davis L, Wimsatt LA (2010) Depression, stigma, and suicidal ideation in medical students. JAMA 304:1181–1190
3. Kamski L, Frank E, Wenzel V (2012) Suicide in medical students: case series. Anaesthesist 61:984–988
4. Hawton K, van Heeringen K (2009) Suicide. The Lancet 373:1372–1381
5. Schernhammer E (2005) Taking their own lives – the high rate of physician suicide. N Engl J Med 352:2473–2476
6. Jurkat HB, Reimer C, Schroder K (2000) Expectations and attitudes of medical students concerning work stress and consequences of their future medical profession. Psychother Psychosom med Psychol 50:215–221
7. Voltmer E, Kieschke U, Schwappach DL, Wirsching M, Spahn C (2008) Psychosocial health risk factors and resources of medical students and physicians: a cross-sectional study. BMC Med Educ 8:46

Injuries from Heavy Machinery

7

Hans-Richard Arntz

▶ Head injuries can, as this case shows, very quickly become very dramatic, especially when "heavy machinery" is used. This case also shows that you are not immune to terrible situations as an emergency doctor, which you might assume to be a one-time occurrence, and that you have to relive them again.

Without a doubt, every emergency physician remembers scene calls after several years of service that he or she will never forget. It is especially astonishing when two unusual events happen one after the other, which, moreover, have not lost their horror even after a long period of time.

The first emergency call came in the afternoon on a quiet weekday. The fire department dispatched us with the keyword "serious injury" without further information on the type of injury to a villa area in Berlin. After a few hundred meters of driving with lights and sirens, the fire department reports again with the more detailed information that it should be a neck injury. Of course, a head cinema immediately arises with possible scenarios; one of them is—as I remember—a gaping neck wound after a fall into a glass door, as they are often found in the villas in Berlin—safety glass was not common back then. Hardly has this image been created, the fire department reports again, now with the message that it is a chainsaw injury to the neck. The joint reaction of our physician-manned ambulance team is that it could possibly be a violent crime—at least our hair stands on end at this thought.

Arriving at the scene of the accident, our imagination seems to be confirmed at first: in front of the entrance of the house there are numerous policemen who look a little confused and, when asked what happened or where we can find the injured

H.-R. Arntz (✉)
Charité, University Medicine Berlin, Campus Benjamin Franklin,
Department of Cardiology and Pulmology, Berlin, Germany

V. Wenzel (ed.), *Case Studies in Emergency Medicine*,
https://doi.org/10.1007/978-3-662-67249-5_7

person or persons, silently point to the open front door. When we enter the house, we see a bloody person sitting in a chair in a room behind the hallway; the chair and the carpet underneath are soaked with blood. The person is—recognizable by the gray stubble beard under the blood—an older man with a huge gaping and heavily bleeding wound on the neck and several other cuts lower down on the neck. Despite the proximity to many large blood vessels, a spurting blood loss is surprisingly not detectable. Despite sitting position and massive blood loss, the injured person, as gesturing attempts show, is obviously at least partially conscious. The possibly completely severed trachea hangs down in front of the large wound, with blood flowing into the trachea and apparently also being aspirated. Despite many years as an emergency physician, I have never experienced such a situation.

While I am determined on the one hand to treat the patient's fear of airway obstruction by aspirated blood and hemorrhagic shock as quickly as possible by induction of anesthesia, I also want to know on the other hand how the situation came about. When cleaning the blood-smeared arms in search of a venous access, I notice numerous large scars on both forearms that originate from longitudinal cuts in the arm. This initially seems to suggest that it may be a suicide attempt. After induction of anesthesia, the patient is intubated and ventilated directly into the outwardly hanging trachea and an infusion therapy is initiated. Only now do I notice other policemen in the room who, after "forced" questioning, point to a half-standing, terror-stricken and petrified-looking older woman who seems to be clinging to the wall. As it turns out, this is the patient's wife, who discovered the situation and first alerted the fire department, which then alerted the police in addition based on the description of the situation. When we ask what happened, the woman silently points to a blood-smeared power saw (so-called "cut-off grinder") lying on the ground with which the patient apparently tried to cut his own throat. However, after the first cut attempt on the neck, which fortunately did not open the carotids, the power saw apparently fell out of his hand. The request to the policemen to help us with the transport of the seriously injured person ends with a typical complication for the following hectic situation when a policeman's boot gets caught in the monitor cable and infusion line, resulting in a loss of the venous access. The new venous access is quickly found despite the blood-smeared arms and the patient can be brought to the hospital after pre-notification for anesthesia and ENT without further incidents. After primary treatment in the emergency room, the patient is operated on immediately, allowing the continuity of the trachea to be restored.

The patient's central problem and his determination to end his life even by using extreme violence against himself are of course not solved by this. The prognosis for such structured and aggressive suicide attempts is generally critical because the probability of success increases with the number of initially failed violent self-destruction attempts [1]. The extent of violence in this sad case makes survival seem more like a miracle anyway, since the large arteries in the neck were only narrowly missed. Intensive psychiatric therapy is of course necessary afterwards; however, I have no knowledge of its results.

Now one thinks that one would experience similar things—if at all—only after a longer period of time, but far from it: Hardly 4 weeks after this terrible deployment, I am again alarmed as the on-call emergency physician at the EMS helicopter on a warm summer afternoon with the keyword "severe injury" to a construction site in Berlin. I can't believe my ears when I hear the additional information "Chainsaw injury in the face". During the approximately 10-minute flight, we of course develop the most terrible ideas about the situation that awaits us.

We find a young worker at the emergency site who has been lying on a blanket by his colleagues as part of first aid. You can see a wide wound that was partially torn off by the chainsaw links at the edges, which ran from the inner right eye corner, near the nose, over the right cheek, split the upper lip and also injured the lower lip and parts of the chin. It is not clear whether there were also injuries to the eye; just as unclear is whether there were deep jawbone fractures or injuries to the row of teeth. What happened? The worker was not sawing from top to bottom as usual when working with the chainsaw on wooden beams, but setting the saw under the beam and sawing it up. When the saw passed through upwards, there was a sudden uncontrolled movement of the approximately 50 cm long saw blade towards the unprotected face of the worker with the described injury consequences. The entire protective equipment of the injured consists only of safety shoes and leather gloves—unfortunately he has dispensed with safety clothing and a helmet with integrated face protection despite the danger.

Since the severity of the injury cannot be determined exactly on site, the young man is conscious and despite clearly high blood loss, circulatory stability seems not to be life-threatening. At the emergency site, we are particularly happy to be able to forego intubation of the airway in order to secure it, as it cannot be ruled out that a necessary strong mouth opening and traction on the lower jaw during laryngoscopy could lead to additional injuries. After sterile wound coverage, insertion of a venous cannula with infusion of a crystalloid solution and sufficient analgesia for the treatment of severe pain, the logical transport destination in view of the complex injury pattern and the specialist disciplines required for further treatment (Ophtalmology, ENT, maxillofacial surgery, plastic surgery) is a hospital of maximum care with our EMS helicopter in order to avoid time losses. With the now possible exact determination of the exact extent of the injuries with optimal examination conditions under anesthesia, it turns out that the young man has had enormous luck in misfortune: the eyeball and the tear duct are uninjured, as is the row of teeth; only the oral cavity is open. Otherwise, only soft tissue injuries are present, but also nerve lesions to a lesser extent, so that only a temporary impairment of facial expression is to be expected. Almost 2 weeks after the event, the patient can be discharged home with a result that is also satisfactory from a cosmetic point of view.

Discussion

It is amazing what curious mechanisms people come up with for a suicide, but it seems to simply correlate with access to the method. In a country like the USA with approximately 200 million firearms in private households, the risk of dying from a firearm suicide is 10 times higher than in a household without a firearm [2]. Physicians, on the other hand, tend to poison themselves with drugs when they attempt suicide because they have easy access to it and know the mechanisms of action [3]. However, what is much more important in the first case is to keep a cool head in the face of the dramatic situation and not to worsen the situation with imprudent therapy approaches—unfortunately there are a number of cases in which, for example, patients have died as a result of botched airway management, who had survivable injuries [4].

The second case shows with what everyday carelessness work is also carried out with dangerous tools, which again and again leads to serious injuries. The mechanism of injury in our patient is typical for chain saw injuries [5], as well as injuries up to amputations of the lower extremities. Careless handling of the regulations, for example the statutory accident insurance for protective clothing and injury prevention (www.dguv.de), among other things specifically when handling chain saws, certainly does not always end as successfully as in our case. By the way, forester's offices often offer very recommendable, usually inexpensive or even free courses for the correct protection and the safe handling of chain saws for private individuals. As much as one wonders about the carelessness of the injured construction worker, so much is everyday carelessness in the life of an emergency medical service evident: EMS employees or emergency physicians who appear for duty in sneakers, ride motorcycles without helmets, run into burning houses without protective equipment or assume when treating injured people on the highway that they will be seen well by other road users. While accidents with physician-manned ambulances that occur in practically every emergency medical center are only discussed in the local press, accidents with helicopter EMS are also analyzed in the scientific literature [6, 7]. All participants in an emergency medical team should address careless behavior and try to prevent it.

7.1 Conclusion

Injuries to the face and neck cause very rapid and severe blood loss; the balance between shock and airway management must be very carefully considered in order to avoid further blood pressure drops and/or respiratory disaster.

References

1. Giner L, Jaussent I, Olie E, Beziat S, Guillaume S, Baca-Garcia E, Lopez-Castroman J, Courtet P (2014) Violent and serious suicide attempters: one step closer to suicide? J Clin Psychiatry 75:e191–e197
2. Miller M, Hemenway D (2008) Guns and suicide in the US. N Engl J Med 359:989–991

3. Schernhammer E (2005) Taking their own lives – the high rate of physician suicide. N Engl J Med 352:2473–2476
4. von Goedecke A, Herff H, Paal P, Dörges V, Wenzel V (2007) Field airway management disasters. Anesth Analg 104:481–483
5. Riefkohl R, Georgiade GS, Barwick WJ (1986) Chain saw injuries to the face. Ann Plast Surg 16:87–89
6. Baker SP, Grabowski JG, Dodd RS, Shanahan DF, Lamb MW, Li GH (2006) EMS helicopter crashes: what influences fatal outcome? Ann Emerg Med 47:351–356
7. Hinkelbein J, Spelten O, Neuhaus C, Hinkelbein M, Ozgur E, Wetsch WA (2013) Injury severity and seating position in accidents with German EMS helicopters. Accid Anal Prev 59:283–288

Blood Pressure Crisis

8

Martin Dünser

▶ This case very clearly shows that a good diagnosis should always also take into account the symptoms and the general condition of the patient before the gaze wanders to the monitoring. This is indeed an important accompanying diagnostic parameter, but by no means the only one.

I am just on night duty and am immersed in the thick medical history of a patient who has been treated on our intensive care unit for weeks, when I am called to admit a patient. An 82-year-old man with fever and a dramatic deterioration in his general condition is brought to our emergency department. Despite several underlying health conditions (arterial hypertension, coronary heart disease with myocardial infarction, chronic heart failure with moderately reduced ejection fraction, non-insulin-dependent diabetes mellitus), the patient lived independently with his wife at home. He is sufficiently resilient for everyday life with only minor restrictions (climbing stairs). Two days ago, the patient developed unspecific illness symptoms with general weakness, became subfebrile and finally febrile (on arrival at the emergency department: 38.9 °C (102 °F)). When the patient was confused this morning after waking up, his wife alarmed the EMS, which brought the patient to the emergency department. The clinical examination does not reveal any indications of focal neurological deficit, neck stiffness, suspicious pulmonary rales, abdominal guarding, joint pain or infective skin changes. A right-sided flank pain and a 3/6 systolic murmur over the Erb's point are conspicuous. With the absence of peripheral endocarditis signs and turbid urine with the detection of leukocytes (+ + +), erythrocytes (+ +, eumorphic) and positive nitrites, the provisional

M. Dünser (✉)
Department of Anesthesiology and Critical Care Medicine, Kepler University Hospital, Linz, Austria
e-mail: Martin.Duenser@kepleruniklinikum.at

V. Wenzel (ed.), *Case Studies in Emergency Medicine*,
https://doi.org/10.1007/978-3-662-67249-5_8

diagnosis of "sepsis with urinary tract infection" and probably "pyelonephritis" is formulated. Differential diagnosis cannot rule out endocarditis. Laboratory analysis shows leukocytosis with left shift (17% neutrophils and toxic granules) and severe thrombocytopenia (67 g/l). After obtaining microbiological cultures, empirical antibiotic therapy is initiated with an aminopenicillin. A renal ultrasound does not show any evidence of obstruction of the renal pelvis or renal calyx system. The patient presents somnolent. He is oriented to person and situation, but does not know what day it is or where he is. His skin is cool and shows a re-capillarization time of 5 s. as well as a skin mottling over the knee. The neck veins are not congested and peripheral venous filling (e.g. on the back of the hand) is reduced. Even manual compression of the liver bed over 10 s. does not lead to dilation of the neck veins. The heart rate is 110/min and the arterial blood pressure 75/30 mmHg. After fractionated administration of 1.5 l crystalloid fluid, the patient shows good peripheral perfusion. His skin becomes warm, the re-capillarization time normalizes to values around 3 s and the skin mottling disappears. The neck veins are visible in supine position 2 cm above the jugulum. Hepatojugular reflux is still not induced. Although the heart rate has dropped to 95/min, the blood pressure remains low at mean arterial blood pressures of 45 mmHg. Much too low compared to the international recommendations of the sepsis societies. Although the nurse at the bed is pleased about the course of the increasingly awake patient, I cannot share this enthusiasm at all. The blood pressure is simply too low! A vasopressor is needed! I start a norepinephrine infusion with the goal of raising the mean arterial blood pressure to values around 65 mmHg. Shortly after the start of the infusion, the blood pressure starts to rise as desired and I return to my medical history. When I reassess the patient after 2 h, the nurse reports that, in order to achieve the desired mean arterial blood pressure, she had to increase the norepinephrine to 0.2 µg/kg/min. The patient is no longer as responsive as before and begins to fidget with his catheters uncoordinatedly. The hands and feet are again cool and the skin mottling over the kneecaps is again clearly visible. The heart rate has risen to 115/min and the diuresis has completely ceased during the last hour. Obviously, the patient is just "slipping" into a severe septic shock. I ask the nurse to continue to administer fluid boluses. Just before the morning handover, the patient is agitated and wants to get out of bed. The lactate has risen to 8 mmol/L, the fingers are already blue and the diuresis is now completely gone. The norepinephrine dose has to be increased to 0.41 µg/kg/min. This will result in mean arterial blood pressure values between 60–70 mmHg in order to save what is left of the kidney from sepsis! I start a dobutamine infusion and change the antibiotic to a carbapenem. Exhausted, I report the mentioned patient with progressive severe shock to the experienced intensive care physician during the morning handover. With the bad feeling that I have done everything right, but still overlooked something, I leave the hospital. When I come back to the ward the next morning, I immediately look for the patient who has been on my mind until then. Expecting to find an intubated, hemodynamically unstable patient on renal replacement therapy, I am surprised when I find a conscious patient. Pleased but also a little disbelieved, I shake his hand and introduce myself. He reacts promptly, smiles and I shake his warm, well-perfused hand in greeting. The experienced colleague comes up to me, smiles and shows me the course of yesterday's events using the automatic computer records. Immediately after taking over, he had performed a transthoracic echocardiography and seen that the ejection fraction of the left ventricle was severely impaired and the patient had a relevant mitral valvel insufficiency. Therefore, he gradually reduced the norepinephrine infusion. Although the blood pressure fell back to the initial values of 45 mmHg mean arterial blood pressure, diuresis improved and lactate fell. I am completely astonished when a sodium nitroprusside infusion, a potent but short-acting vasodilator, is started and the mean arterial blood pressure even begins to rise slowly. This is associated with a further increase in diuresis. In the afternoon of the same day, I receive the microbiological finding of the urine or blood culture, in which a pansensitive *E. coli* was detected in each case. I de-escalate the carbapenem to an aminopenicillin. The patient is discharged to the ward in good general condition 2 days later.

Discussion
As described in Ohm's law, blood pressure is the product of flow and resistance or, physiologically simplified, of cardiac output and vascular resistance. Although arterial blood pressure is often equated with blood flow and, thus, with organ perfusion in practice, studies of the past 10 years have impressively shown that this assumption is not always correct [1, 2]. In several clinical studies, no relationship was found between blood pressure and microcirculation or other markers of organ perfusion. Furthermore, clinical studies have shown that a large proportion of patients with sepsis still have impaired tissue perfusion after norepinephrine-mediated increase of mean arterial blood pressure to target values of 65 mmHg [3, 4]. The example of our patient is particularly impressive because the sepsis-induced circulatory dysfunction is worsened by poor left ventricular function and relevant mitral valve insufficiency. But that's just how it is in clinical practice - not only in individual cases, but if you look closely, in a majority of cases! Both cardiac pathologies are known and it is also known that they usually deteriorate with an increase in left ventricular afterload. That is what happened in our patient's case. After initial improvement due to fluid therapy, the liberal and blood pressure value-controlled norepinephrine infusion eventually led to a significant deterioration of the patient's condition, who then showed almost all signs of systemic hypoperfusion. As a result of the alpha-mediated vasoconstriction, the vascular resistance and, thus, the afterload of the left ventricle were significantly increased. This led to a critical reduction of cardiac output due to deterioration of pump function and increase of mitral insufficiency. Even the small beta-mimetic effects of norepinephrine or administration of dobutamine could not change this. Although blood pressure increased to recommended values of 65 mmHg under this false therapy for the patient, tissue perfusion (peripheral perfusion, lactate concentration) and organ function (urine output, confusion) deteriorated dramatically. Only after stopping

the norepinephrine infusion was the afterload reduced again, which caused the pump function to increase and the mitral valve insufficiency to decrease. Although this led to a decrease in mean arterial blood pressure, it was accompanied by an increase in cardiac output and tissue perfusion. Therapy with sodium nitroprusside further reduced vascular resistance and, thus, led to an additional increase in cardiac output. The improvement of (organ) perfusion under this therapy was evident from the normalization of peripheral perfusion, the re-establishment of urine output and the decrease in lactate concentrations.

8.1 Conclusion

This patient's case changed my view of hemodynamic therapy for acutely and critically ill patients significantly. It led me back to the textbooks of physiology, taught me to understand the real meaning of cardiac afterload, and demanded that I keep my promise to learn echocardiography from scratch. Today I am convinced that blood pressure at low values is mostly a marker of disease severity and must under no circumstances be set to arbitrary target values with noradrenaline, in blind faith in a number on the monitor. The clinical picture and the examination of the patient is still the essential decision-making basis for controlling circulatory therapy in hemodynamically unstable patients, despite all technical innovations. Norepinephrine for the treatment of arterial hypotension should only be used in exceptional cases (critical coronary, aortic and/or carotid stenosis, right heart failure) if there are clinical signs of increased vascular resistance. The underlying problem, which is caused by systemic hypoperfusion in many cases of sepsis, must be treated causally and as quickly as possible. Furthermore, the understanding that there is only a small relationship between blood pressure and tissue perfusion taught me that many patients can be in severe shock despite normal or even increased blood pressure and have a life-threatening tissue hypoperfusion. So let's focus primarily on the patient, his/her clinical signs and only then on the monitor [5] in the future!

References

1. De Backer D, Creteur J, Preiser JC et al (2002) Microvascular blood flow is altered in patients with sepsis. Am J Respir Crit Care Med 166:98–104
2. Lima A, van Bommel J, Sikorska K, van Genderen M et al (2011) The relation of near-infrared spectroscopy with changes in peripheral perfusion in critically ill patients. Crit Care Med 39:1649–1654
3. Rady MY, Rivers EP, Nowak RM (1996) Resuscitation of the critically ill in the ED: responses of blood pressure, heart rate, shock index, central venous oxygen saturation, and lactate. Am J Emerg Med 14:218–225

4. Lima A, van Bommel J, Jansen TC et al (2009) Low tissue oxygen saturation at the end of early goal-directed therapy is associated with worse outcome in critically ill patients. Crit Care 13(5):S13
5. Dünser MW, Takala J, Brunauer A et al (2013) Re-thinking resuscitation: leaving blood pressure cosmetics behind and moving forward to permissive hypotension and a tissue perfusion-based approach. Crit Care 17:326

Buried Under Concrete Slabs

9

Bernd Domres and Norman Hecker

▶ Natural disasters pose great challenges for external rescue forces; especially in developing countries. The local treatment options usually do not correspond to the treatment strategies that are common in western industrialized countries. Although doctors in developing countries often have outstanding improvisational talent, they can benefit from our help, for example in treatment algorithms.

A mother has just come home from work and is setting the table for dinner. Suddenly there is a growling, then deafening noise: walls and floors of the apartment shake and sway, windows and dishes shatter, the ceiling of the apartment and the multi-storey building collapse. Our patient is buried deep under the rubble, a heavy concrete slab is lying on her left arm and leg.

An earthquake of magnitude 7.2 on the Richter scale, with the hypocenter at a depth of 17 km (10.6 miles) and 25 km (15.5 miles) southwest of Port-au-Prince in Haiti, destroyed large parts of the capital inhabited by more than 2 million people; more than 200,000 residents lost their lives and more than 1.8 million people were homeless [1]. Due to the chaotic conditions, a precise registration and identification of the victims was not possible, so that the number of victims could only be estimated. About 250,000 apartments and 30,000 businesses were destroyed; the damage amounted to more than 5 billion Euro or US Dollars, which exceeded Haiti's gross domestic product- extrapolated into Germany this would be an earthquake damage of 2500 billion Euro or US-Dollars. This makes Haiti 2010 the worst earthquake in the history of North and South America, as well as the worst

B. Domres (✉)
Foundation of the German Institute for Disaster Medicine, Tübingen, Germany

N. Hecker
Department of Emergency Medicine, Protestant Hospital, Gelsenkirchen, Germany
e-mail: hecker@evk-ge.de

V. Wenzel (ed.), *Case Studies in Emergency Medicine*,
https://doi.org/10.1007/978-3-662-67249-5_9

earthquake of the twenty-first century worldwide. At first, relief workers mainly come from neighboring countries such as the Dominican Republic and Cuba, before some days later also relief workers from Europe arrive; the US Navy sends a hospital ship and an aircraft carrier off the coast of Haiti to transport injured people by helicopter to non-destroyed hospitals.

It is not until January 15, 3 days later, that rescue workers manage to rescue our patient from the rubble and only by amputating the already lifeless arm with a tourniquet applied using a concrete cutter. The femur of the left leg, which was trapped under the concrete slab for 3 days, has suffered an oblique fracture and, with severe swelling, paresthesia and motor paralysis, shows the signs of a manifest compartment syndrome. Our patient is taken to a hospital by the rescue team to have her left leg amputated there because of the compartment syndrome with beginning crush syndrome. Our team of doctors from the Humedica organization from Kaufbeuren, Germany works in the hospital.

Discussion

Disasters do not follow personal schedules. They happen unexpectedly. If you are on the other side of the world from a disaster, it usually starts with text messages on your cell phone. So it was in January 2010: "Earthquake in Haiti, sending first team. Tonight from Munich, feedback in 2 h, duration 14 days. Second team will be set up within the next 2 days."

In this specific case, this message means the immediate personal decision about one's own availability. For civilian forces, this is an enormous burden, because only a few relief organizations have the financial resources to provide a pool of experts who are always available. Essentially, these are established physicians and specialist nurses as well as specially trained organizers who are available on a humanitarian and voluntary basis. They often provide essential medical supplies such as drugs, spinal needles and vital monitoring or surgical equipment from personal initiative.

The arrival in a disaster area in the immediate response is anything but a trip planned in detail, but rather resembles a parachute jump. It usually leads by plane as close as possible to the crisis area in order to achieve ground contact there together with the official cargo of the relief organizations and the personal luggage. It can then be helpful to carry personally provided medical aid as hand luggage, as medical materials have a tendency to be delayed at customs—especially if entry into the disaster area leads through a third country. In the case of Haiti, large parts of the aid taken along by the team were held in the Dominican Republic for 2 days.

Disasters, especially earthquakes, often destroy infrastructure dramatically. In the case of Haiti, the earthquake mainly affected the region around the capital (Port-au-Prince) and thus the center of resistance to disasters of the entire nation. Here were personnel and materials from police, fire brigades, medical facilities and the United Nations. Also, the region is the central axis of the transport connection to and from abroad. Therefore, among the more than 200,000 dead and injured of the earthquake were central forces of disaster prevention.

In 2010, the journey continued from the airport, often over long distances, in jeeps, buses or trucks. In the destroyed region, sometimes only rugged terrain and impassable side roads were left. The actual main roads were destroyed or blocked by refugees. Such a difficult way can take days despite only a few 100 km (62 miles). The actual mission for the teams is at this point still a thought game, but with the arrival in the mission area the work begins.

Here new challenges and unexpected hurdles await. Rarely are the conditions on site similar to the clinical reality at home. Volunteer civilian teams then orient themselves to the known clinical structures of their homeland and organize the available infrastructure accordingly. The teams are inventive, flexible and well trained in individual medicine, but usually not practiced in teamwork and limited in their resources.

The indication for amputation in the case of manifest compartment syndrome, as in our patient's case, was made too often after the earthquake in Haiti, in our opinion. After the patient's admission, the examination by the Humedica team showed that the prognosis of saving the leg was actually promising. The Humedica team made the indication for dermo-fasciotomy of the left leg and for surgical stabilization of the femur fracture after initiation of intensive care measures for the treatment of shock and impending crush syndrome such as shock treatment (potassium-deficient electrolyte infusion via 2 peripheral IV lines), diuresis (furosemide), acidosis buffering (sodium bicarbonate, until the urine pH is above 6.5), correction of hyperkalemia (glucose infusion in combination with regular insulin), thrombosis prophylaxis, as well as therapy of cardiac arrhythmias (300 mg amiodarone). Fortunately, this made dialysis unnecessary, which would otherwise have been difficult to organize [2]. According to the experience of an Israeli army medical team, depending on the position of the earthquake debris in Haiti, up to 25% of the rescued patients had a crush syndrome, of which in turn 0.5–25% developed acute renal failure. If one considers the many thousands of injured and that more than half of the patients with acute renal failure need dialysis and thus have extremely good survival chances, one can estimate how many people initially survived after a catastrophic earthquake like in Haiti, but died due to the lack of treatment options for acute renal failure [3]. Our patient recovered quickly and was happy that she did not lose her left leg after losing her left arm.

9.1 Conclusion

Our finding that the indication for amputation was too rigorously made in the case of a compartment syndrome after the Haiti earthquake prompted us to develop an algorithm for the indication of surgical measures in the case of impending and manifest compartment syndrome in the event of a disaster. If a compartment syndrome is impending, a dermo-fasciotomy should be carried out within the first six hours if possible; if more than six hours have elapsed, a re-evaluation should be carried out every four hours. In the case of a manifest compartment syndrome within the first six hours, it depends on whether an irreversible vascular or nerve damage, multiple trauma, age over 18 years, diabetes or muscle necrosis is also present; if so, an amputation should be carried out, if not, a dermo-fasciotomy and possibly a necrosectomy can be performed. If the compartment syndrome manifests itself more than six hours after the event and only one extremity is affected and there is no crush syndrome, a dermo-fasciotomy and possibly a necrosectomy may be sufficient. However, if in addition to the compartment syndrome there is sepsis, several extremities are affected, a crush syndrome, no dialysis possibility, a multiple trauma, diabetes or age over 75 years, an amputation is usually the only option.

References

1. Rice MJ, Gwertzman A, Finley T, Morey TE (2010) Anesthetic practice in Haiti after the 2010 earthquake. Anesth Analg 111(6):1445–1449
2. Vanholder R, Gibney N, Luyckx VA, Sever MS (2010) Renal disaster relief task force. Renal disaster relief task force in Haiti earthquake. Lancet 375(9721):1162–1163
3. Bartal C, Zeller L, Miskin I, Sebbag G, Karp E, Grossman A, Engel A, Carter D, Kreiss Y (2011) Crush syndrome: saving more lives in disasters: lessons learned from the early-response phase in Haiti. Arch Intern Med 171(7):694–696

Emergency on the Fairground

10

Hans-Richard Arntz

▶ Emergency calls are difficult when, from apparently complete health, a life-threatening situation suddenly and unexpectedly arises without any clearly recognizable or comprehensible cause, such as an accident. The present case impressively shows how an intervention can occupy us even after the end of the service, indeed even many years later.

On an afternoon around 4:00 pm, our physician-manned ambulance is alarmed at the Benjamin Franklin Hospital with the keyword "sudden unconsciousness". The emergency address is a ride at the German-American Folk Festival on Clay Avenue in Berlin-Zehlendorf. We take on the approximately 4 km (2.5 miles) long alarm drive relatively relaxed, assuming that we have to take care of a smaller, typical alcohol-related problem at such a folk festival. However, the first difficulty arises already upon arrival, at the several hundred meters / yards long, and partly fenced outdoor area of the large festival grounds with several entrance possibilities. Since we were not told which entrance to choose, we take the nearest entrance and ask the security guard there for the exact emergency site, of which he "of course" knows nothing. While the security guard is informed by radio, we learn from the EMS control center that it is a cardiopulmonary resuscitation attempt of a child or adolescent. Meanwhile, the security guard has found out that the emergency site is practically at the other end of the festival grounds. So we have an alarm drive across the whole square in front of us, right through the numerous pressing people. Some of the festival visitors apparently hold the physician-manned ambulance with siren and blue lights on the festival grounds for an entertainment gag and behave accordingly understandingless. Meanwhile, we are

H.-R. Arntz (✉)
Charité, University Medicine Berlin, Campus Benjamin Franklin,
Department of Cardiology and Pulmology, Berlin, Germany

© The Author(s), under exclusive license to Springer-Verlag GmbH, DE, part of Springer Nature 2023
V. Wenzel (ed.), *Case Studies in Emergency Medicine*,
https://doi.org/10.1007/978-3-662-67249-5_10

increasingly under pressure in view of the information available to us and the slow progress.

Finally, after certainly more than 15 min after alarm activation arriving at the emergency site, we get the following picture: a larger number of curious people have gathered at the emergency site, which are pushed back by the also arrived police. On the ground lies a boy aged 11 years. The ambulance team, which had arrived earlier, had taken over the cardiopulmonary resuscitation attempt from 2 first aiders and had laid the child on a stretcher. As it turns out, both first aiders are companions of the boy: one an uncle, who is a paramedic by profession, the other rescuer is the spouse of the boy's mother. Both have started the resuscitation attempt immediately after the detection of the circulatory arrest at the exit of the ride. The rescue team that arrived before us had already defibrillated 2 times with the semi-automatic defibrillator—ventricular fibrillation still exists. After an immediate 3rd shock with maximum energy output, ventricular fibrillation is eliminated, but there is an asystole in the ECG.

The further standard measures, such as orotracheal intubation and venous access, can be carried out easily during continuous thoracic compression; however, injection of epinephrine initially has no effect. After several minutes of continuing cardiopulmonary resuscitation, re-injection of 1 mg epinephrine after further consistent thoracic compression over several minutes shows effect in the form of a coordinated rhythm with initially weak, then better palpable pulse and increase in end-expiratory carbon dioxide concentration. When stabilization appears to be achieved, we make preparations for transport, but in the monitor we first observe an increasing bradycardia with rapid transition into a new asystole. The new resuscitation attempt does not result in a circulatory reaction within the next 15 min. Since asystole persisted despite all efforts, we finally discontinued resuscitation at 16:50 h, after a total of 35 min aggressive resuscitation. Every emergency physician knows this: it is all the harder to accept death, the younger the deceased is. It often becomes an event that one never forgets when the death of a child also occurs from apparently complete health without any clearly recognizable or comprehensible cause, such as an accident.

Discussion

What had happened? The ride is a small roller coaster "for the whole family" with a maximum speed of 50 km/h (31 mph) and partly tight curves. At the end of the ride, the passengers in each car automatically shot a Polaroid photo for remembrance. The entire facility had been checked and released by the TÜV (a technical supervision organization in Germany) a few days earlier for technical and electrical safety. The 11-year-old victim was sitting on the front seats of one of the 4-seat cars secured by bars next to his 10-year-old sister. An adult sitting behind the siblings had observed that the boy apparently collapsed during the ride. In fact, the Polaroid photo taken at the end of the ride showed the boy slumped, with his head leaning against his sister's chest. The boy's uncle, a paramedic, immediately recognized the situation and started cardiopulmonary resuscitation immediately after the child was freed from the car. Meanwhile, the ride operator had alarmed the fire brigade and police. A thorough examination of the normally developed deceased child showed no physical abnormalities, no injuries and in particular no power marks that would have been possible with the electrically operated ride system. The ride was closed immediately and examined by an expert who found no defects. The questioning of the boy's uncle and the mother's spouse did not reveal any indications of an acute or chronic illness. The boy had not complained of any problems before the ride, on the contrary they had a lot of fun.

Since I was asked to deliver the sad news of the sudden and completely unexpected death of her son to the mother of the deceased child, I tried to combine this difficult task with a questioning of possible abnormalities in the medical history of the deceased and the family medical history; e.g. with regard to unexplained fainting spells or even deaths at young ages or in children. With the understandable excitement caused by the ride on the roller coaster as a potential trigger of an arrhythmia, one had to think of a genetically determined predisposition to malignant arrhythmias, such as the Long-QT-Syndrom or catecholaminergic polymorphic tachycardia [1]. We were particularly sensitized by an unfortunate course in 2 young sisters [2]. Of the sisters, the younger one died suddenly with initial ventricular fibrillation and unsuccessful resuscitation attempts. In the medical history, there was talk of a suspicion of epilepsy with repeated collapse states. The autopsy showed no pathological findings. A few weeks later, the slightly older sister of the deceased also died after initially successful resuscitation in ventricular fibrillation: she also had a suspicion of epilepsy. On the monitor of the initially surviving person, we saw Torsade de Pointes and the typical signs of Long-QT-Syndrome on the intensive care unit and in the ECG. The family medical history revealed further cases of unexpected early death, including in children, and affected persons with a history of collapse and the evidence of a genetic aberration typical for Long-QT-Syndrom [2].

In our case, however, the mother's survey did not result in any suspicious clues; not even in the family of the divorced husband. Both children had also grown up without any health problems so far. At least I was able to convince the mother to have an ECG registered for herself, her daughter and as many other close relatives as possible—but I have not heard anything about the results. The body of the deceased child was confiscated and a forensic autopsy was ordered. According to the information of the autopsy physician, this did not reveal any pathological findings or clues that could explain the sudden death of the 11-year-old boy. My urgent request, also for preventive medical reasons, to have a molecular genetic examination carried out, was rejected for cost reasons and lack of competence. However, it was subsequently possible to learn from the Institute of Legal Medicine that ECGs had been registered in some family members, but these had been unspectacular. So the question of a possible cause of death in this tragic case of an unexpected sudden death remained unanswered—in particular, it was not clarified whether disorders such as the Brugada syndrome or the polymorphic rhythm disorders that can be seen under load in the case of adrenergic polymorphic ventricular tachycardia (APVT) were possible causes that could only be recognized with Ajmalin and pharmaceutical provocation. The thought of this unanswered question oppresses me to this day. Perhaps it would have been possible to have the deceased child and, if necessary, also relatives examined genetically via the mother. All known, genetically determined potentially fatal rhythm disorders can indeed be successfully treated by influencing the lifestyle (avoiding stress), pharmacologically (ß-blockers in Long-QT syndrome or APVT) and in the case of documented high-risk or survived cardiac arrest by implantation of an implantable defibrillator.

10.1   Conclusion

In unexplained deaths in infants, adolescents and young adults, a genetically determined cardiac disorder must be considered. The family history is essential (further unexplained deaths, atypical epilepsy, recurrent collapse?).

Simple additional tests, such as a 12-channel ECG, can be helpful, but are not particularly reliable, as in the case of a long QT syndrome. Dangerous QT prolongations only become manifest in some patients—especially in women—under the influence of certain drugs; e.g. a variety of antiarrhythmics, macrolide antibiotics, antidepressants and other psychopharmaceuticals, antimalarials, etc. A careful drug history is therefore also important. If a Brugada syndrome is suspected, an Ajmalin provocation test is necessary. Stress tests can also be helpful in uncovering the propensity for malignant rhythm disorders.

At the latest in the case of additional suspicious cases in the family history, targeted diagnostic steps should be taken in relatives for the sake of potentially life-saving prophylaxis, and the need for a genetic test in a younger patient with an unclear cause of death should be emphasized.

References

1. Beckmann MB, Pfeufer A, Kääb S (2011) Erbliche Herzrhythmusstörungen. Dtsch Ärztetbl 108:623–634
2. Witzenbichler B, Schulze-Bahr E, Haverkamp W, Breithardt G, Sticherling C, Behrens S, Schultheiss HP (2003) An 18 year old patient with anti-epileptic therapy and sudden cardiac death. Z Kardiol 93:747–753

Inferno on the Highway

11

Peter Hilbert-Carius

▶ The case described demonstrates how quickly the neglect of basic emergency medical/tactical measures can lead to a very confusing situation. An accident scene with multiple casualties always presents the first-responding rescue team with special challenges.

On a clear, warm, and cloudless summer morning, the team of an EMS helicopter receives a call from the rescue dispatch center for an incident on a highway with the alarm code "traffic accident with multiple vehicles, vehicles on fire, ground-based EMS and fire department on site". It is obviously a classic secondary alarm by the ground-based EMS for quick patient transport, so the assumption of the EMS helicopter crew. Already during the approach to the accident scene, a black column of smoke can be seen from several kilometers away, and during the landing approach it is possible to see that 2 trucks and 3 cars were involved in the accident. The trailer of the truck that rear-ended the first truck and a car are on fire. So it can be assumed that there are several injured people to be cared for.

The EMS helicopter lands at a safe distance from the accident scene and near the two ambulances that are already on site. After landing, the EMS helicopter's emergency physician goes to the emergency physician who is already on site and is to take over the role of the lead emergency physician in order to obtain information on the number of patients, the assessment category, and the further procedure. At this point, the first-responding emergency physician is treating a patient in one of the two ambulances. In response to the question of how many injured people there are and which the EMS helicopter crew should take care of,

P. Hilbert-Carius (✉)
Department of Anesthesiology, Critical Care, Emergency Medicine and Pain Therapy,
Bergmannstrost BG-Hospital, Halle/Saale, Germany
e-mail: Dr.PeterHilbert@web.de

V. Wenzel (ed.), *Case Studies in Emergency Medicine*,
https://doi.org/10.1007/978-3-662-67249-5_11

the first-responding emergency physician replies that he does not know and that he now has to take care of this patient. This leads to appropriate irritation on the part of the EMS helicopter crew. This is followed by the question of whether an assessment and possible triage have taken place, to which the answer is "no". It is the impression that any further questions would not lead to any gain in information. So far, it has not been possible or not possible for the rescue forces on site to get a quick overview of the situation, the number of injured people, and the assessment category of the injured people. Since this has not been possible, the EMS helicopter team takes over the assessment, which is more difficult than expected. There are obviously 5 vehicles involved in the accident, as mentioned above, a truck trailer and a car are on fire, while the fire department is just extinguishing the fire. The highway has already been completely closed in the direction of the accident by the police, while traffic in the opposite direction is still normal. The patient being treated by the first-responding emergency physician is apparently the truck driver of the second truck that rear-ended the first truck, whose trailer is on fire. The driver of the first truck, which the other vehicles rear-ended, is apparently uninjured. Any help comes too late for the 4 occupants of the first car that rear-ended the burning truck (sedan); they are already burned. A second car (medium-sized station wagon), which had also been set up, can be saved by the fire department before ignition. The car's airbag had triggered. But there are no more occupants in this car and on the back seat is an empty child seat (Group 1, 9–18 kg (20-40 lbs) age group 1 to approx. 4 years). Initially, it is not possible to determine who was sitting in the car and whether a child was an occupant or not. A fifth vehicle, also a car (medium-sized sedan), which apparently had tried to avoid the rear-end collision and in the process had hit the guardrail on the shoulder, is only slightly damaged. The airbag of this vehicle had not triggered. The driver is next to his vehicle and looks unharmed. So far, the situation is: one injured and one uninjured truck driver, one obviously uninjured car driver, 4 burned, dead car occupants and one vehicle with a child seat involved in an accident, of which no occupants are known so far. When children are involved in an accident, emotions are always a little more tense, the colleagues of the highway police already on site and some firefighters are asked by the EMS helicopter crew to search for and find the occupants of the car. After a short time, the completely frightened older driver of the car can be found. She had the child seat for her grandson in the car, which she had previously handed over to her daughter, and she was therefore alone in the car. This leads to the relief of all participants, since there is apparently no injured child. The patient has some small abrasions on her forehead and nose, which may be due to the airbag. After the end of the inspection and forwarding of this information to the local EMS control center, the injured truck driver, who is now immobilized by means of a vacuum mattress and Stiff Neck, is flown to a regional trauma center. The frightened driver of the second car with the child seat is also transported to a regional trauma center in the company of the ground-based emergency physician. The diagnostics carried out here for the truck driver reveal a thoracic trauma with lung contusion, rib fracture 2-4 left and transverse process fracture of the thoracic vertebrae 2 and 3. The driver of the car has no other injuries besides her abrasions and the psychological trauma.

Discussion
The case described demonstrates how the neglect of basic emergency medical/tactical measures can quickly lead to a very confusing situation, even though there were actually enough rescue forces and EMS personnel available at the accident site. An accident situation with several injured people always poses special challenges for the first-responding rescue team [1]. In such situations, it is necessary to deviate from the usual individual medical care, as one is used to from emergency medical services, i.e.: one injured/sick person, one treatment team. In this case, it is about assessing how many injured/sick people are present, how severe the injury/illness is, in order to alarm an appropriate number of suitable rescue vehicles and possibly a leading emergency physician and organizational leader subsequently. Only when sufficient rescue forces are available should treatment of each individual injured person begin. With damage situations involving several injured people, initial individual medical criteria cannot be applied [2]. Rather, it is a matter here of setting priorities and initially treating the patients who have a high probability of survival. In order to make this clear, the patients are classified into 5 sighting categories as part of the assessment and each category is assigned a certain color, which also represents the treatment priority:

- In sighting category 1 (color red), there are seriously injured people with vital endangerment.
- Sighting category 2 (color yellow) includes seriously injured people without vital endangerment.
- Sighting category 3 (color green) refers to lightly injured patients.
- Sighting category 4 (color blue) is intended for severely injured people without a chance of survival (dying).
- In the last sighting category 5 (color black), dead patients are classified.

In the situation described above, the first arriving physician would have had to gain an overview of the situation. After appropriate inspection, it would have been clear early on that 4 patients of inspection category 5 (black), one patient of inspection category 2 (yellow) and one patient of inspection category 3 (green) were at the accident site. In this context, it would have become clear more or less quickly that the originally alarmed rescue forces (2 ambulances, one physician-manned ambulance and the fire brigade) were sufficient for the management of the accident. However, the reordering of the EMS helicopter appears to be fundamentally sensible in traffic accidents or unclear damage situations. Although the case described was far from representing a mass casualty incident, emergency physicians should still deal with the circumstances of such a scenario in advance, as it usually comes unexpectedly and then basic knowledge is of advantage. Even if it was not a mass casualty incident, the case still shows how important it is to gain an initial impression of an emergency situation. To obtain this, a structured approach is helpful. "Structured" means in this case: observe self-protection, inspect and categorize the accident and the patients, and after the first inspection, decide whether the available rescue resources are sufficient (as in this case) or not. If they are not sufficient, the appropriate rescue resources must be requested from the rescue control centre.

For the case of a real mass casualty incident, some algorithms have proven themselves in the treatment strategies [3, 4], which can not be discussed any further at this point.

11.1 Conclusion

In addition to self-protection and the provision of a quick overview in the form of an inspection, it must be decided promptly whether the available resources are sufficient or, if not, the appropriate forces must be requested. This task and the management of medical care initially belong to the tasks of the first arriving physician.

References

1. Beck A, Bayeff-Filloff M, Kanz K-G, Sauerland S (2005) Algorithm for mass casualties at the accident site: A systematic review. Notf Rettungsmed 8:466–473
2. Beneker J, Marx FA, Mieck F, Reinhold T, Ekkernkamp A (2014) Großunfälle – Erfahrungen aus drei Realeinsätzen. Notarzt 30:206–217
3. Paul AO, Kay MV, Hornburger P, Kanz KG (2008) Mass casualty incident management by mSTaRT. MMW Fortschr Med 150:40–41
4. Wolf P, Bigalke M, Graf BM, Birkholz T, Dittmar MS (2014) Evaluation of a novel algorithm for primary mass casualty triage by paramedics in a physician manned EMS system: a dummy based trial. Scand J Trauma Resusc Emerg Med 22:50

Collapse While Doing Barn Work

12

Martin Dünser

> What is common in the hospital is often common—if you hear hoofbeats, you should look for horses, not zebras—this often facilitates the diagnosis, say American colleagues. But: There is always an exception to this. You can assume a statistical number, but you must not forget that there is always a "plus-minus" or simply a zebra.

Thursday, late morning on one of our intensive care units. The transfer reports are written, the rounds are almost finished. Everything looks like lunch before the postoperative admissions come from the OR. But then the emergency room reports: a patient after cardiopulmonary resuscitation is to be taken over. The 43-year-old lady collapsed while doing farm work. According to the emergency physicians, lay resuscitation was started quickly, which was continued by paramedics after a short time. When the emergency physician arrived, there was pulseless electrical activity. Given the young age of the patient and the lack of previous illnesses (the only thing that can be raised: syncope 1 week before the event), cardiopulmonary resuscitation was continued for a total of 60 min. After the 13th injection of epinephrine, asystole converted to ventricular fibrillation, which could be successfully defibrillated. Despite the prolonged cardiopulmonary resuscitation attempt, circulation is stable. With an uneventful ST segment in the ECG, no regional wall motion disorders or signs of right heart dilatation in the echocardiogram as well as a bland skull CT (with contrast agent to exclude a basilar thrombosis), a conduction disorder with preexisting left bundle branch block is the most likely cause of the circulatory arrest. The "nice" thing about recordings of patients

M. Dünser (✉)

Department of Anesthesiology and Critical Care Medicine, Kepler University Hospital, Linz, Austria

e-mail: Martin.Duenser@kepleruniklinikum.at

V. Wenzel (ed.), *Case Studies in Emergency Medicine*, https://doi.org/10.1007/978-3-662-67249-5_12

after cardiopulmonary resuscitation is the standardized procedure that the international guidelines give us: 1) targeted temperature management 2) placement of appropriate IV accesses, 3) sedation and maintenance of therapeutic hypothermia for 24 h, 4) slow rewarming and 5) stopping of sedation usually 30–36 h after admission. This is followed by this moment of uncertainty: the hope of awakening a neurologically intact patient, which is often disappointed by the patient's lack of response and makes way for the sad, almost nihilistic feeling of having to make the diagnosis of hypoxic brain damage again. Often this phase of anxious waiting is interrupted earlier, namely by a cerebral seizure—just like our patient. A few minutes after the sedation was stopped, the patient developed a generalized tonic-clonic seizure, which could be terminated by the injection of lorazepam, but then turned into a non-convulsive status epilepticus. This can only be interrupted after 48 h by an antiepileptic triple therapy (levetiracetam, valproic acid, lacosamide). The further EEG findings show what everyone has already feared: slow theta-delta activity without reaction to exogenous stimuli. The medianus-SSEP-evoked potentials can only be derived on one side with a clear reduction in amplitude. All these electrophysiological findings correspond to the clinical picture of the patient, who remained deeply comatose with preserved brainstem reflexes. After the MRI diagnosis of generalized diffusion disorders in almost all cortex areas and the brainstem ganglia as well as the certification of a dismal prognosis by the neurological consultant, the relatives who have been previously informed about the poor course of the disease are confronted with the option of discontinuing therapy. However, the religious multi-member family cannot make such a decision to discontinue therapy and wishes to continue intensive care therapy including tracheotomy and PEG feeding tube placement. In the certainty that the patient will develop a (persistent) vegetative state, repeated family meetings are held in which the lack of possibilities for neurological recovery is pointed out. One of these always open and friendly conversations took place as follows. I hear myself saying the following sentence: "If it were my relative, I would not want her to survive in such a state." The deep belief of the family is ultimately stronger than all our medical certainty of an irrecoverable hypoxic brain damage. 22 days after admission, the patient is transferred to neurorehabilitation. The feeling that we have not done everything to protect the patient and, above all, the relatives from the fate of a vegetative state, prevails among us for some time until—about 2 weeks later—the neurologist reports surprised and pleased at the same time that the patient would begin to react to her environment. A short time later she is contactable and can leave rehabilitation for the home environment after 2 months. The only demonstrable neurological deficit at discharge is a cortical visual disturbance. The patient has since visited us twice with her family and even reported that she can return to her work on the farm. And both times I apologized for my statement, because we have never been so far off in the assessment of the neurological prognosis.

Discussion

Therapeutic temperature management after cardiopulmonary resuscitation significantly improved neurological prognosis [1]. At the same time, however, the assessment of neurological prognosis became significantly more complex compared to the time before the introduction of therapeutic hypothermia [2]. While in the past clinical signs, such as a myoclonic or epileptic status, could predict a poor outcome after cardiopulmonary resuscitation with a false-positive rate of almost 0% [3], after the introduction of therapeutic hypothermia even previously reliable signs for a poor neurological outcome could hardly be used anymore. Thus, the probability of functional recovery could only be estimated by interpretation of the neurophysiological test results together with the repeated clinical examination. Only over time and through the analysis of large international databases did we learn to better estimate the neuroprognosis after cardiopulmonary resuscitation with subsequent therapeutic hypothermia [4]. According to the current state of knowledge, certain combinations of clinical-neurological, electrophysiological and laboratory findings indicate a very poor recovery potential (defined as death, vegetative state or severe physical disability) [4, 5]. This puts the false-positive rate back in comparable ranges as before the introduction of therapeutic hypothermia.

12.1   Conclusion

The course of the patient described also raises doubts about the findings of a false-positive rate in predicting neurological recovery. Nevertheless, this does not contradict the literature, which describes a false-positive rate (i.e. the chance of a good outcome for a bad one) of 0% on average for the observed finding constellation, but gives a confidence interval of 0-3% [4–6]. This means that a small number of all patients who have these symptom constellations still have a good neurological prognosis. There is currently no indication of how to identify these individual patients. Maybe there are subtle clinical hints that we have not yet recognized or interpreted, but which nevertheless provide such valuable information that no therapy should be discontinued. If there were such clinical or other signs, we obviously overlooked them in the patient described.

References

1. Arrich J, Holzer M, Havel C et al (2012) Hypothermia for neuroprotection in adults after cardiopulmonary resuscitation. Cochrane Database Syst Rev 9:CD004128
2. Rossetti AO, Oddo M, Logroscino G et al (2010) Prognostication after cardiac arrest and hypothermia: a prospective study. Ann Neurol 67:301–307

3. Young GB (2009) Clinical practice. Neurologic prognosis after cardiac arrest. N Engl J Med 361:605–611
4. Sandroni C, Cavallaro F, Callaway CW et al (2013) Predictors of poor neurological outcome in adults of cardiac arrest: a systematic review and meta-anylsis. Part 2. Patients treated with therapeutic hypothermia. Resuscitation 84:1324–1338
5. Oddo M, Rossetti AO (2014) Early multimodal prediction after cardiac arrest in patients treated with hypothermia. Crit Care Med 42:1340–1347
6. Kamps MJ, Horn J, Oddo M et al (2013) Prognostication of neurologic outcome in cardiac arrest patients after mild therapeutic hypothermia: a meta-analysis of the current literature. Intensive Care Med 39:1671–1682

Fall into Icy Water

13

Luise Schnitzer

▶ In the case of an accident, in addition to the questions of injury, the triggering mechanism is also important in order to be able to treat not only the symptom, but also the cause. Sometimes the injury and mechanism are completely evident, sometimes you have to ask persistently- as in this case.

Our emergency call reads: "Person in water". It is a cold November day, it is getting dark. Passers-by have discovered a person in a canal and alerted the fire brigade. The person is floating still in the water and does not move. A thrown life-buoy is already floating in the water, but has drifted too far from the person. The rescue forces from the ambulance have re-alarmed a rescue boat from the fire bri-gade and are now trying to help the person floating in the water by throwing a rope to her, but without success. After about 8 minutes the team from the rescue boat, which is quickly launched, reaches us. They quickly approach the person in the water and call her. But to our surprise, the patient now stirs and swims away from the rescue boat. It takes a while until the crew finally reaches the person in the water and can pull her into the boat with combined forces. The woman, com-pletely soaked and hypothermic, sits on the stretcher- we take off her wet clothes and wrap her in a warm blanket. The physical examination does not reveal any serious findings: her circulation is stable, blood pressure 120/70 mmHg, the heart rate 57/min, the body temperature 35.4 °C (95.7 °F). After the woman has recov-ered a little, she can, still shivering, answer our many questions.

She is unmarried and has no close relatives. She had a beautiful job that allowed her a sufficiently good pension. She has few, but good friends, most of

L. Schnitzer (✉)
Medizinische Klinik für Kardiologie und Charité University Medicine Berlin, Campus Benjamin Franklin, Department of Cardiology and Pulmology, Berlin, Germany
e-mail: l.schnitzer@gmx.de

V. Wenzel (ed.), *Case Studies in Emergency Medicine*,
https://doi.org/10.1007/978-3-662-67249-5_13

them her age, but also already a little frail and cared for by their families. She has always been healthy and fits, but now her strength is failing and the care of her household is becoming more and more difficult. Since she does not want to be a burden to anyone, she has decided to take her own life. Having always been an enthusiastic swimmer who had taken part in many competitions in her youth, she felt the water to be the right element for her purpose. She wanted to drown- and yet she was very surprised that this did not work. Whenever she had submerged, the impulse to new swimming strokes had been stronger and she had hoped to get tired and drown eventually if she stayed in the water long enough. But then the rescue boat and the doctor appeared... During the story, the patient becomes more and more lively, she doubts herself and is also very pleased with the care and interest she receives from the entire rescue team. With a mischievous smile she then remarks that she is glad to have left her dentures at home- because: "I can still use them quite well!"

The patient is being treated further in the hospital, special measures are not required for moderate hypothermia. Several conversations with the social service then lead to the patient being subsequently accommodated in a nursing home. There she quickly settles in and is still happy today that her suicide attempt was not successful.

Discussion

The rescue of a patient after a failed suicide is a sad reason for an intervention, which—at least in this case—has its humorous sides and has ended well. This makes it easier for me to have helped a patient in an apparently hopeless situation. Suicide is always a doubly sad occasion and occasionally I can't get rid of the thought of whether I am really acting in the patient's interest when I try to save him. This is all the more true for an older person who, in their mind, have lived their life and now come to the conclusion that it is enough. Nevertheless, we must not forget that often in this situation it is not in the foreground that the patient is really "tired of life", but that external factors—such as the desire not to be a burden to anyone—are often motivation for the suicide attempt. And we have to keep in mind that by simply providing attention, information and human interest these factors can be easily changed—whether by accommodation in a caring nursing home, by establishing contacts with relevant aid organizations or by therapeutic measures. In many suicides—whether by young or old people—it turns out afterwards that the triggering factors could have been controlled from the outside, but the patient either did not have this help available or did not have the courage or the strength to ask for it. Of course, one cannot prevent a suicide-determined person from attempting suicide; but many suicidal patients work on their situation successfully after a failed suicide attempt and have a normal life expectancy afterwards.

A study by the WHO shows: the older people become, the higher the risk that they will commit suicide. In 2011, 10,000 people took their own lives in Germany, the proportion of people over 60 years was 40%. In a Swedish study [1], family conflicts, serious illnesses, loneliness and a depressive illness are mentioned as reasons why older people in particular want to commit suicide. M. Wehr also finds these fears in her diploma thesis [2]. These fears are understandable because they concern our independence and our human dignity.

13.1 Conclusion

More people die in Germany every year from suicides than from traffic accidents. The main reasons for a suicide are described in the Gotland study [3]; in this study it could be shown that diagnosed depressions are often treatable and that the suicide rate can be significantly reduced as a result—90% of suicides have a psychiatric diagnosis or a corresponding illness. N. Erlemeier [4] comes to the following conclusion in his book:

We cannot promise people to free them from their suffering in old age; but offering to accompany them in their distress would make a lot of things much easier.

References

1. Waern M, Rubenowitz E, Wilhelmson K (2003) Predictor of suicide in the old and elderly. Gerontology 49:328–334
2. Wehr M (2007) Suizid im Alter. DIPLOMARBEIT im Fachhochschulstudiengang Soziale Arbeit. Otto-Friedrich-Universität, Bamberg
3. Rihmer Z, Rutz W, Pihlgren H (1995) Depression and suicide on Gotland. An intensive study of all suicides before and after a depression-training programm for general practitioners. J Affec Disord 35(4):147–152.
4. Erlemeier N (Jahr) Suizidalität und Suizidprävention im höheren Lebensalter (Taschenbuch 29. Sep 2011), Kohlhammerverlag.

Choking Attack in Nursing Home

14

Peter Hilbert-Carius

▶ How should one behave if one cannot be sure that something else is available than what one would consider right in the first place in an emergency situation? The present case deals with an important problem that rescue forces can encounter and for which there is no universal solution approach.

On a Sunday morning, the crew of an EMS helicopter is alerted by the rescue control center with the mission report "unconscious person". The scene call goes to a nursing home on the outskirts of a large city. During the flight to the scene call site, which takes about 5 min, it is not possible to obtain any further information, except that an ambulance has also been sent to the scene call site. The landing of the EMS helicopter is possible directly next to the nursing home and from the air it can be seen that the ambulance has already arrived. When the doctor arrives at the patient, the following picture emerges: A man of about 70 years is lying on the ground and is cyanotic. The first rescue team that arrived is already performing cardiopulmonary resuscitation by means of chest compressions and mask ventilation with reservoir bag and oxygen application. The patient is already connected to the EKG monitoring, in which asystole can be seen in all derivations. While cardiopulmonary resuscitation is still ongoing, the following is to be learned from the nursing staff: The patient had breakfast and suddenly complained of coughing and shortness of breath; shortly afterwards he became unconscious. Furthermore, there is a past medical history of diabetes and a high blood pressure. The patient has a living will and does not want hospital treatment. When asked whether the patient is a "bedridden nursing case", this is denied and it is stated that the patient is still

P. Hilbert-Carius (✉)
Department of Anesthesiology, Intensive Care, Emergency Medicine and Pain Therapy,
BG Trauma Hospital Bergmannstrost, Halle/Saale, Germany
e-mail: Dr.PeterHilbert@web.de

V. Wenzel (ed.), *Case Studies in Emergency Medicine*,
https://doi.org/10.1007/978-3-662-67249-5_14

very fit and takes care of himself to a large extent in the nursing home. During the short collection of the history of the disease, an intravenous access is placed during ongoing cardiopulmonary resuscitation by the physician. This is connected to a balanced crystalloid infusion solution and 1 mg epinephrine is injected. Shortly afterwards, individual ventricular complexes can be seen in the EKG. The patient was now intubated with an 8.0 mm ID tube under vision, the intubation site corresponding to a Cormack/Lehane Score II and the intubation being carried out without problems. However, it turned out that when pushing the tube forward at about 18 cm dental row, a clear resistance could be felt and the tube could not be pushed further against the resistance . When trying to ventilate via the tube with the ambu bag, an extremely high ventilation resistance is observed, which also persists after slight withdrawal; no sufficient thoracic excursion can be achieved. Since the tube is safely in the trachea (intubation under vision) and the history of the disease points to a possible aspiration, the following further procedure is decided: The breathing connector of the tube is removed, the tube is connected to the fingertip of the suction hose of the suction pump and the tube is removed under maximum suction of the suction pump.

In this way, 2 slices of ham, which are sucked directly into the tube, can be removed. After readjusting for intubation, 2 more slices of ham can be removed with Magill forceps. The patient can then be intubated again without difficulty and the tube can be inserted without resistance. Even ventilation with bilateral ventilation of the lungs is now possible. After tube fixation and ventilation adjustment, asystole is again shown in the ECG. After another injection of 1 mg epinephrine and continuation of cardiopulmonary resuscitation with 100% oxygen ventilation via the endotracheal tube, a spontaneous circulation with clearly palpable carotid pulse can be recorded about 2 min after epinephrine injection. In the ECG, supraventricular and ventricular heartbeats are initially shown, which convert into a sinus rhythm a short time later. End-tidal carbon dioxide rises from 15–18 mmHg during cardiopulmonary resuscitation (after the successful second intubation attempt) to 35–40 mmHg during the regained spontaneous circulation. The patient is already cooled prehospitally with appropriate cooling packs, sedation with diazepam and fentanyl is initiated and the patient is transported by the EMS to a hospital of maximum care. Here the patient is circulatory stable, without catecholamines and with a sinus rhythm. The cardiac diagnostics ordered in the hospital shows a moderate coronary heart disease without massive stenosis or myocardial infarction. The patient can be extubated on the 4th day after the event and is transferred to a rehabilitation facility after 3 weeks in the hospital. At the time of transfer, the patient is awake, oriented, but still slowed down in cognitive performance.

Discussion

The case described demonstrates several important aspects that should be considered in emergency medicine. First, you encounter an elderly patient with a circulatory arrest and an advance directive. Here the question arises as to whether initiation or continuation of cardiopulmonary resuscitation is justified at all? This question is basically difficult to answer and there is no "panacea" for this. Only a few arguments should be listed here, which, in the opinion of the author, also speak in favor of the initiation or continuation of cardiopulmonary resuscitation in this or a similar situation. The event was observed and the time window until the start of cardiopulmonary resuscitation by the EMS team was short, which generally appears to be favorable for the prognosis, although the initial asystole observed in the ECG rather suggested an unfavorable prognosis [1]. The patient was elderly, but according to the statement of the nursing staff still independent and active. From the past medical history and the existing long-term medication, no indications of limiting underlying diseases emerged. The existence of a possible advance directive should also not be generally taken as an occasion not to initiate cardiopulmonary resuscitation. Furthermore, in a resuscitation situation, one will probably barely have time to deal with the advance directive, to read it and to decide whether the directive now also covers the present situation. As already mentioned above, there is no "panacea" with regard to the initiation and/or termination of resuscitation and this is an extremely situation-related, individual and partly difficult process. Even the current guidelines initially recommend starting cardiopulmonary resuscitation in principle, in order to then possibly discontinue it if the rescuers are presented with an advance directive that limits the treatment [2]. In the situation described (elderly patient with existing advance directive), we were glad in retrospect that we had consistently carried out cardiopulmonary resuscitation.

A second important aspect that is illustrated by the case is the fact that circulatory arrest does not necessarily have to be of cardiac origin in the older patient population. In addition to the purely cardiac causes, easily treatable reversible causes should always be considered. These causes are summarized with the 4 Hs "hypoxia, hypovolemia, hypo-/hyperkalemia, hypothermia" and the 4 Ts "tamponade (cardiac), toxins, thrombosis (coronary and pulmonary), tension pneumothorax" [3]. The present case impressively shows that in this patient the cause of the circulatory arrest was of hypoxic nature due to massive aspiration. That this is not so rare is shown by the work of Sakai et al. [4], which showed that 466 (19.8%) of 2354 patients with aspiration developed circulatory arrest. If it is possible to eliminate hypoxia in a timely manner through the initiated resuscitation measures, the prospects for successful resuscitation are often very good. So it could also be shown in the already mentioned work of Sakai et al. that if it was possible to eliminate airway obstruction by using the Magill forceps preclinically, this was a predictor of survival with good neurological outcome [4]. The case described here confirms this impressively. The anamnestic finding to be elicited from the history that the patient suddenly developed a strong coughing attack with subsequent dyspnea during breakfast and became unconscious a short time later must necessarily lead to the suspicion of a possible aspiration. Also from this point of view, it would not be justified to interrupt ongoing cardiopulmonary resuscitation attempt knowing that there may be an easily treatable reversible cause for the circulatory arrest.

The aspiration described in the present case must be described as massive and unusual. Four slices of ham so deep into the trachea that were not visible during laryngoscopy for intubation, while the described Cormack/Lehane II score only allowed a view of a small subglottic part of the tracheal posterior wall, is already amazing. This shows how intense the patient's breathing efforts must have been that such a high negative pressure was developed that the ham reached so deeply into the trachea. Since no foreign body was visible during laryngoscopy, the primary use of the Magill forceps to remove the described airway obstruction made no sense. Therefore, only 2 alternatives were left in the situation when it was clear that ventilation via the lying tube was not possible. On the one hand, one could have tried to push the tube further with a lot of force to push the airway obstruction into the right main bronchus in order to enable ventilation via the left lung. However, since the resistance felt on the tube seemed very high, this variant was not chosen in order to proceed according to the method described above. The removal of the tube under suction turned out to be successful and can be considered for similar cases. The described procedure has already proven itself several times during the author's emergency and intensive medical activities.

14.1 Conclusion

The existence of an advance directive does not necessarily mean the renunciation of life-saving measures, especially if they are associated with a high success rate. In the case of massive aspiration of solid food into the trachea, as described, the possibility of removing foreign bodies by continuous suction on the tube and slowly removing the tube should be considered.

References

1. Andrew E, Nehme Z, Lijovic M, Bernard S, Smith K (2014) Outcomes following out-of-hospital cardiac arrest with an initial cardiac rhythm of asystole or pulseless electrical activity in Victoria. Australia. Resuscitation 85(11):1633–1639
2. Lippert FK, Raffay V, Georgiou M, Steen PA, Bossaert L (2010) Ethics of resuscitation and end of life decisions. Notf Rettungsmed 13:737–744
3. Deakin CD, Nolan JP, Soar J, Sunde K, Koster RW, Smith GB, Perkins GD (2010) Adult advanced life support of the European Resuscitation Council Guidelines for Resuscitation Notf Rettungsmed 13:559–620
4. Sakai T, Kitamura T, Iwami T, Nishiyama C, Tanigawa-Sugihara K, Hayashida S, Nishiuchi T, Kajino K, Irisawa T, Shiozaki T, Ogura H, Tasaki O, Kuwagata Y, Hiraide A, Shimazu T (2014) Effectiveness of prehospital Magill forceps use for out-of-hospital cardiac arrest due to foreign body airway obstruction in Osaka City. Scand J Trauma Resusc Emerg Med 22:53

Traffic Accident in Construction Area

15

Sven Wolf

> ▶ There are techniques and procedures that are not in any textbook, but come from the years- or decades-long experience of other emergency physicians. This case shows that these skills can save lives in the crucial moment.

Late at night, a truck with a trailer collides head-on with a low-floor articulated bus on an empty run in a construction area on a highway. Both drivers are seriously injured and trapped, but responsive. 2 physician-manned ambulances, 2 ambulances, 2 rescue squads and a crane truck are dispatched. After lighting up a suitable landing site, an EMS helicopter is also dispatched later. Both vehicles collided half-overlapped head-on at the level of the vehicle drivers with a penetration depth of about 1 m. The bus driver is trapped in the leg/pelvic area, circulatory stable, prima vista there is a closed left upper arm fracture, a closed right lower leg fracture and a decollement injury on the left thigh. The truck driver is trapped in the left shoulder, thorax and pelvic area, the left arm is stuck up to the shoulder (acromioclavicular joint) in the destroyed roof structures of the bus. Prima vista there is a forehead wound, and a head trauma (Glasgow Coma Scale 13; conditionally responsive), an open left arm injury (at the level of the upper arm, below the destroyed bus roof, a constant trickle of mixed arteriovenous blood is visible as an indication of a fulminant vascular injury); the blood pressure is 110/70 mmHg, the heart rate is 118 and oxygen saturation is 95% at room air.

The initial assessment of the medical-technical dispatch assumes that a technical rescue and medical treatment of the bus driver is urgent, but without any significant expected problems. The vascular injury on the left arm of the truck driver is not accessible at all; there is therefore no possibility of manual haemostasis or

S. Wolf (✉)
Department of Emergency Medicine, DIAKOVERE Friederikenstift, Hannover, Germany
e-mail: drsvenwolf@web.de

V. Wenzel (ed.), *Case Studies in Emergency Medicine*,
https://doi.org/10.1007/978-3-662-67249-5_15

application of a tourniquet. A crash rescue is therefore absolutely indicated; however, a non-critical, quick separation of both vehicles is not possible due to the unstructured impact situation in the area of the truck/bus roof/arm of the driver—the approximate time to remove the bus roof in the area of the arm by the fire department is about 30–45 min.

After technical rescue and the medical first aid of the circulatory stable, responsive and oriented bus driver, the transport takes place with an ambulance and physician-manned ambulance to a hospital of specialized care. The treatment of the truck driver is initially carried out with two 14-G-accesses (venous) on the right arm (2000 ml Ringer solution) and immobilization of the cervical spine. With increasing circulatory depression (blood pressure 90/00 mmHg, heart rate 135, oxygen saturation 95% with 2 l/min O_2 over nasal cannula), an indication for intubation of the sitting patient is made, which succeeds easily with 15 mg midazolam and 0.2 mg fentanyl. After a short discussion and weighing of the medical-technical options (uncontrolled, inaccessible bleeding in a trapped patient), the emergency physician decides on an open-surgical intervention in the area of the left arm. After a spray disinfection on the left shoulder, the attachment of a sterile gauze cloth to the clavicle fails at first due to the lying cervical spine orthosis (stiff-neck); the sterile gauze cloth is then stuffed behind the thorax. After palpation of the clavicle and the lateral boundary of the M. sternocleidomastoideus, a 5 cm long longitudinal skin incision is made with the scalpel directly on the cranial clavicle edge lateral to the sternocleidomastoideus with division of platysma/fascia. Subsequently, the artery is blunt-prepared or "drilled" with the index finger dorsally-medially-caudally to the pulsating A. subclavia/brachialis up to the first rib; then the artery is compressed with the finger on the underlying first rib. As a result, the uncontrolled bleeding stops immediately. This position is maintained by the emergency physician for 23 min, during which he has to change his finger 3 times due to cramping during the technical rescue. The circulatory situation remains stable at a low level. A perfusion pump with arterenol is prepared, but is not used in the course. After the stepwise separation of the destroyed roof parts with hydraulic scissors and spreader, in addition to a closed ellbow dislocation fracture, a deep incision wound at the transition from the medial proximal upper arm to the anterior axillary line is revealed, which was caused by a torn metal edge of the roof. The mixed bleeding from the A. and V. brachialis can then be controlled axially against the humerus head up to the hospital by manual compression with the thumb or the fist. The previously attempted placement of a tourniquet almost in the area of the anterior axillary line fails due to the anatomical conditions. After another 19 min, the patient is technically freed and rescued with a spineboard over the work platform. The subsequently ordered EMS helicopter then transports him to a hospital of maximum care about 50 km (31 miles) away with continuously stable circulatory conditions. After initial surgical reconstruction of the two vessels and parts of the brachial plexus, a year later a good outcome is shown with moderate neurological, motor-sensitive deficits of the left arm.

Discussion

The surgical intervention of the emergency physician described resembles more an abstract "live-saving-procedure" of war surgery [3, 5], because of a problem in the middle of one of the world's best rescue service infrastructure. Undoubtedly, the emergency physician was faced with an extreme "ultima ratio situation" [4]. Within the curriculum of our emergency medical training and in interdisciplinary, partly international course formats such as ATLS, easy-to-use decision paradigms for prehospital procedures and emergency room management are conveyed; for example "stop the bleeding", "life before limb", and "treat first what kills first". And therefore we also know about the relatively high mortality of open, arterial extremity injuries [2]. The emergency surgical access to a central extremity artery described above is not found in any standard textbook or surgical procedure atlas. It was conveyed to our emergency physician as part of a DSTC© course [Definitive Surgical Trauma Care; ATLS© and DSTC© courses are offered in German-speaking countries, for example, by the German Society for Trauma Surgery (www.dgu-online.de)]. Based on the charismatic Johannesburg trauma surgeon Kenneth D. Boffard, the 3-day course is basically aimed at all acute-surgical physicians [1]. Due to the tactical focus, doctors of the German armed forces are often found in the auditorium who are planned for deployment abroad. Sometimes unconventional tips and tricks are conveyed theoretically and practically on the basis of a very large experience with blunt, stabbing and gunshot wounds. Most of the "skills", such as the emergency room thoracotomy with temporary control of a perforating cardiac injury using a commercially available catheter, require surgical basic skills and at least the infrastructure of an emergency room. Tourniquet and also emergency amputations are repeatedly discussed and described in individual case studies in our rescue service landscape [6, 7]. In the specific individual case, after surgical intervention, the central extremity artery was compressed manually against the first rib. This "live-saving procedure" is and remains an extreme example; it will probably never find its way into our regular curriculum of emergency medicine. And yet it was a brave ultima ratio decision without any recognizable alternatives in this case. During the post-mission debriefing, the question arose as to why, if an emergency surgical intervention was already carried out, the artery was not "clamped" immediately? This was not done in the specific individual case for 3 reasons: In the immediate anatomical vicinity of the A. subclavia is the brachial plexus and the pleural dome, the light or visibility hardly makes this possible, and the anatomical site is at least 5 cm below skin level and, even with optimal surgical conditions (Langenbeck hook, suction device, 2 experienced assistants, operating light, vessel instruments, blood coagulation), is only difficult to represent.

## 15.1	Conclusion

It is generally also worth looking beyond the "horizon" in EMS. Certainly, ideas for alternative bleeding control are by no means as essential as knowledge in alternative airway management. But even if only one EMS patient were to benefit from it within 10 years, one would be on the winning side!

References

1. Boffard KD (2007) Manual of definitive surgical trauma care. Hodder Arnold, London
2. Gümbel D, Naundorf M, Napp M, Ekkernkamp A, Seifert J (2014) Diagnosis and management of peripheral vascular injuries. Unfallchirurg 117(5):445–459
3. Hodgetts TJ, Mahoney PF, Evans G, Brooks A (2002) Battlefield advanced life support. J R Army Med Corps 152(2 suppl):4–64
4. Holcomb JB, Champion HR (2001) Military damage control. Arch Surg 136:965–966
5. Husum H, Gilbert M, Wisborg T (2000) Save lives, save limbs: life support for victims of mines, wars and accidents. Third World Network, Penag
6. Johansen K, Daines M, Howey T, Helfet D, Hansen ST Jr (1990) Objective criteria accurately predict amputation following lower extremity trauma. J Trauma 30:568–572
7. Raines A, Lees J, Fry W, Parks A, Tuggle D (2014) Field amputation: response planning and legal considerations inspired by three separate amputaions. Am J Disaster Med 9(1):53–58

Unconscious Woman in Bathroom

16

Martin Messelken

▶ In this case, hypothermia management is in the foreground. The situation at the scene plays a decisive role here, which the EMS and the emergency doctor expect here. Drawing the right conclusions from the circumstances is also associated with obstacles in this case.

Relatives alarm the emergency physician and EMS on a January morning. The emergency physician and his team find a deeply unconscious, poorly dressed obese young woman lying on her back on the tiled floor of an unheated bathroom; she had last been seen 13 h earlier. Because of a depression, she was in psychiatric treatment and had already had several suicide attempts behind her. In the bathroom there are empty boxes of Atosil−, Saroten− and Ludiomil tablets (tricyclic antidepressants), which again suggest a drug overdose. All clinical findings point to an intoxication with severe hypothermia (an exact temperature measurement is not possible): medium-sized unreactive pupils, bradycardia and weak central pulse as well as gasping. With extremely gentle treatment, for the therapy of insufficient respiration and for the protection against aspiration, the patient is quickly intubated and mechanically ventilated. Because of the prevailing circulation centralization, a central venous access must be placed, which succeeds without problems in the V. jugularis interna. However, the subsequent intravenous injection of atropine does not work. Since the EMS was not prepared at that time to use external heat, the patient is only wrapped in blankets and transported to the ambulance under avoidance of active and passive movement in order to be transported to the internally led intensive care unit of the nearby hospital. There, a deep rectal measurement of the body temperature results in 24.9 °C (76.8 °F).

M. Messelken (✉)
Bad Boll, Germany
e-mail: m.messelken@gmail.com

V. Wenzel (ed.), *Case Studies in Emergency Medicine*,
https://doi.org/10.1007/978-3-662-67249-5_16

With continuation of the controlled ventilation, a gradual rewarming takes place, which is carried out by means of a hemofiltration technique and a gastric lavage with 50 l (13 gallons) of warm water. In this way it is possible within 24 h to wean and extubate the patient quickly without any problems by balancing a fluid balance and restoring cardiovascular and thermal homeostasis. Apart from a short passage syndrome, the patient does not show any pathological central neurological symptoms. Since by now also no somatic disorders have occurred and the patient is known in the nearby hospital for neurology and psychiatry due to her past medical history, a transfer is ordered soon [1].

Discussion

For the EMS and the emergency physicians, patients with deep hypothermia always pose a significant problem because the unintentional mixing of core and shell blood during the rescue procedures can lead to the feared rescue death (Afterdrop). Therefore, careful handling of the patient is of paramount importance in all treatments. First and foremost, however, the central body temperature must be determined as early as possible in order to assess the degree of danger. Hypothermia thermometers are available today, but not at that time. Therefore, the severity of the clinical symptoms was the only criterion for the degree of danger. Taking into account the environmental conditions and the clinical findings, a correspondingly deep hypothermia was to be expected. The placement of a central venous catheter under these preclinical conditions is now also assessed differently, since the intraosseous puncture technique is available for efficient drug administration. In principle, however, the injection of cardiovascular drugs is critically seen because of an unpredictable effect in hypothermia.

The handling of such hypothermic patients posed many problems for hospitals at that time, since the sophisticated techniques and technical support for temperature maintenance were (not yet) not routinely available. In this respect, the clinical use and administration of a moderate veno-venous hemofiltration procedure was then and is now an effective and targeted measure. Today, greater emphasis will be placed on the assignment to a suitable hospital, possibly involving the use of air rescue. If cardiac arrest occurs before or during the treatment of hypothermia, immediate resuscitation measures are always indicated, which, with the simultaneous use of extracorporeal support systems, are the preferred option [2].

16.1 Conclusion

Even in our latitudes, life-threatening hypothermia occurs again and again in patients with intoxication by alcohol or drugs. Recognizing a vita minima should not pose a problem, rather it is patients with hypothermia-related symptoms of exhaustion and paralysis. The situation of finding the patient plays a decisive role, which should also make the EMS and the emergency physician think of this differential diagnosis.

References

1. Meßelken M (1986) Tiefe Hypothermie bei suicidaler Tablettenintoxikation. Notfallmedizin 12:379–382
2. Brugger H, Putzer G, Paal P (2013) Accidental hypothermia. Anaesthesist 62(8):624–631

Collapse During Tennis Match

17

Hans-Richard Arntz

▶ This case study shows how important consistent CPR can be, and how surprisingly an emergency can run its course—even years after the event.

The July day is a blisteringly hot day with temperatures of about 39 °C (102.2 °F) in the shade. This does not prevent the then 58-year-old patient from playing tennis outdoors on a sports field in Berlin. Apart from moderate arterial hypertension, he had never been seriously ill and able to perform until that day. In the early afternoon, at the time of the greatest heat, the EMS helicopter is alerted with the keyword "resuscitation"—it is a follow-up alarm by an ambulance of the Berlin fire brigade already on the scene. After a few minutes of flight time, we already overlook the situation from the air: the ambulance crew is in the process of resuscitating a person lying on the tennis court. Two other people are standing next to them. A landing possibility is available on the court near the scene of the incident and is immediately used by our pilot. On arrival at the patient lying on the tennis court in the heat of the sun, we are informed by the firefighters who are continuing to resuscitate (chest compressions, mask ventilation) that they have already defibrillated the patient several times with their automatic external defibrillator without success. After initiating the usual first extended resuscitation measures (orotracheal intubation, venous access via the external jugular vein), we can find out more: the patient suddenly collapsed lifelessly while playing tennis. A physician assistant, who was on a neighbouring court, immediately rushed to help and initiated lay resuscitation with another person. Both persons left the scene shortly after the arrival of the ambulance. It is unclear who alerted the EMS. The patient's

H.-R. Arntz (✉)
Charité, University Medicine Berlin, Campus Benjamin Franklin,
Department of Cardiology and Pulmology, Berlin, Germany

V. Wenzel (ed.), *Case Studies in Emergency Medicine*,
https://doi.org/10.1007/978-3-662-67249-5_17

spouse is sitting in the shade of a tree at the edge of the sports field because she is unable to help.

Discussion

Further measures initially followed the Advanced Cardiac Life Support Guidelines [1]: Epinephrine, repeated amiodarion, renewed attempts at defibrillation, some of which resulted in brief success with demonstrable perfusing very slow rhythm (carotid pulse safely palpable intermittently). However, a blood pressure was only detectable for less than one minute each time and ended in renewed ventricular fibrillation. Spontaneous respiration was not observed. In the desperate situation, an attempt was also made to influence the recurrent ventricular fibrillation with lidocaine, but this was unsuccessful. Another problem proved to be that the entire crew present, drenched in sweat in the sweltering heat of the sun, despite taking turns at thoracic compressions, slowly fell into a state of exhaustion with potential negative effects on the efficiency of the chest compressions. Not only the crew, but also the previously used defibrillator of the ambulance showed signs of exhaustion in the form of increasingly long charging phases until it was ready to defibrillate. After switching to the EMS helicopter defibrillator, we decided to prepare a 12-lead ECG while continuing the above-mentioned measures (i.e. omitting some chest wall leads for the time being) in order to register a complete ECG during one of the next phases with a perfusing rhythm (the missing electrodes were then to be glued on quickly). At this point, the EMS helicopter crew had already been involved in cardiopulmonary resuscitation for 30 min, the ambulance crew for about 40 min. In addition, the estimated time between collapse and arrival of the ambulance was also about 10 min, partly bridged by lay rescuers. In total, the duration of the resuscitation efforts was already approaching 1 h at this point. The status was still characterised by the sequence ventricular fibrillation-defibrillation-occasional short circulatory phases with a conspicuously slow pulse-again ventricular fibrillation. We saw a chance, albeit a small one, of being able to diagnose a recent myocardial infarction with the help of the ECG and stabilise the patient with lysis therapy. At that time, we had seen very promising courses in some freshly resuscitated patients with signs of infarction in the ECG still registered on site—however, no experience in a case like this patient's [2]. Indeed, shortly afterwards, the opportunity for ECG registration presented itself in a period with palpable pulse of just over 1 min duration: the ECG showed the characteristic signs of a fresh inferior myocardial infarction with massive ST-segment elevations in leads II, III and AvF as well as opposing depressions in I and AvL. In addition, there was a total AV block with a ventricular rate of approx. 30 beats/min—the explanation for the strikingly slow pulse already felt beforehand. Systemic thrombolysis therapy with concomitant medication (heparin + aspirin) was then immediately initiated and the resuscitation attempt continued unchanged. After two or three more attempts at defibrillation, a stable, albeit very bradycardic, replacement rhythm was finally established with persistent total AV block visible on the monitor. As the systolic blood pressure was only 70 mmHg, we decided to use external ventricular pacing, which also succeeded stably after some effort. Half buried under the complex but necessary equipment, the patient could then be transported by ambulance to the nearest suitable hospital with invasive cardiology. However, a memorable scene occurred: the patient's spouse had been sitting in the shade at the edge of the sports field during the whole time. As we walked past her with the deeply unconscious ventilated patient on the stretcher, she asked with wide eyes if she could talk to her husband again for a moment. Quite taken aback, I could only tell her that it was not possible now, that her husband had been resuscitated with a very small, but not excluded, chance of survival and told her the destination hospital. After initial standard care, including a passive invasive pacemaker, the course there was really unusual. As the ST-segment elevation had already clearly regressed, coronary acute intervention was not performed (which would certainly no longer be considered optimal nowadays [3]). The ECG, including the V4re lead, also showed ST-segment elevation there as an indication of right ventricular infarct involvement, which was confirmed echocardiographically and also clinically. The patient developed a septic disease on the floor of a left basal pneumonia during already stable circulatory conditions, so that he could only be extubated on day 9. The neurological development was astonishing, especially considering the resuscitation time of about 1 h: the patient only briefly showed minor signs of a transit syndrome with limited retrograde amnesia. A coronarography was only performed 15 days after the event. The findings in the area of the left coronary artery were largely unremarkable and revealed a high-grade concentric stenosis in the area of the distal third of the right coronary artery, which was treated with PTCA without stenting. The echo at discharge showed hypokinesia inferoposterolaterally as a relict of the infarction; all other findings were largely normal. Exercise at 75 W on the ergometer was possible without complaints at discharge. The patient was discharged to a rehabilitation hospital for follow-up treatment.

I was all the more surprised when, a few months later, I received a letter from the patient's spouse on the tennis court, who had meanwhile become his wife. In addition to the pleasant information about the marriage, she reported on a very active life together without a disability. Since then, at intervals of 3–4 months, I have received postcards from the couple from various holiday destinations including reports of skiing holidays etc.—most recently more than 16 years after this happy outcome for all concerned.

17.1 Conclusion

As long as a patient has ventricular fibrillation, they have a chance of survival.

The key to survival is in the hands of potential first responders. Without the energetic initial intervention of the physician assistant and another rescuer, the patient would probably not have survived. That the doctor's assistant or the second person had resuscitation skills is unclear, but probable.

Equally important is the consistent continuation of the basic measures of CPR. Without the obviously optimal performance of CPR by the rescue forces involved, the survival of the patient during a resuscitation attempt lasting approx. 1 h would be almost inconceivable.

The fact that the patient repeatedly developed short phases of palpable circulation was certainly also important for his survival. It is conceivable that at least during some of these e.g. longer phases the "clock was set to 0" again.

Thrombolysis therapy is not generally indicated as an uncontrolled routine during resuscitation [3]. However, it should be considered in certain situations, e.g. in patients who develop an unstable circulation in the meantime. The lysis attempt seems particularly useful in patients in whom it is possible to register a 12-lead ECG and demonstrate ST-segment elevation myocardial infarction (of course, lysis is also the standard therapy for fulminant pulmonary artery embolism in shock or when resuscitation is necessary).

References

1. Wenzel V, Russo SG, Arntz HR, Bahr J, Baubin MA, Böttiger BW, Dirks B, Kreimeier U, Fries M, Eich C (2010) Comments on the 2010 guidelines on cardiopulmonary resuscitation of the European Resuscitation Council. Anaesthesist 59(12):1105–1123
2. Arntz HR, Wenzel V, Dissmann R, Marschalk A, Breckwoldt J, Müller D (2008) Out-of-hospital thrombolysis during cardiopulmonary resuscitation in patients with high likelihood of ST-elevation myocardial infarction. Resuscitation 76(2):180–184
3. Böttiger BW, Arntz HR, Chamberlain DA, Bluhmki E, Belmans A, Danays T, Carli PA, Adgey JA, Bode C, Wenzel V, TROICA Trial Investigators, European, Resuscitation Council Study Group (2008) Thrombolysis during resuscitation for out-of-hospital cardiac arrest. N Engl J Med 359(25):2651–2662

Bus Accident in South Tyrol

18

Hermann Brugger

▶ A bus accident in the mountains can pose a great challenge to the rescue forces and bring unpredictable problems with it. This case also shows how important the prevention of major events is.

When I left Austria and settled in the Pustertal in South Tyrol/Italy, there was no regular emergency medical service in South Tyrol yet, although the number of accidents was shocking. Every day there were serious traffic accidents on the narrow, poorly signposted and unsecured roads, workplace accidents on remote mountain farms, or mountain accidents. Injured people often had to wait a long time for first aid and transport from the mountain valleys to the hospital could take hours. In individual cases, military helicopters were used, which were more suitable as troop carrier than an EMS helicopter. Shortly after my settlement, I started to set up a makeshift emergency medical service with the help of the local fire brigade and trained the best of the fire brigade to be EMS assistants. The men who were used to fire fighting practiced for days in car wrecks, learned rescue techniques, resuscitation measures and the preparation of infusions and intubation, and helped to equip an emergency vehicle for emergency medical care. I was called by telephone during the day from my office and at night from sleep, after a few minutes I was in the EMS vehicle, surrounded by my paramedics from the voluntary fire brigade, a short briefing, then it went to the accident site.

Only a few days after the completion of the training and the beginning of this improvised service, the telephone rings at 2 pm: "This is the fire brigade, motorcycle rider crashed into a gorge. We'll be with you in a minute!" With the deep gorge of the deployment site in front of my eyes, I take my prepared mountain

H. Brugger (✉)
EURAC Research, Institute of Mountain Emergency Medicine, Bozen, Italy
e-mail: hermann.brugger@eurac.edu

V. Wenzel (ed.), *Case Studies in Emergency Medicine*,
https://doi.org/10.1007/978-3-662-67249-5_18

rescue backpack from the storage and put on the protective clothing. In the already waiting EMS vehicle I ask for the first details. Now it says that a car has crashed, further details are unknown. The valley with our deployment site is a deeply cut gorge into the mountains for the drainage of the Dolomites. The road runs winding along the river course, is cut in the rocks along the entire length, without tunnels or other protection against rockfall and avalanches, high above the watercourse. Just before we leave the Pustertal to turn into the valley, the radio message reaches us: "fully occupied long-distance bus 100 m deep crashed, number of accident victims unknown". There are only a few meters left to the entrance to the gorge, where there is no telephone and radio connection anymore: the last chance to make an emergency call to alarm additional forces. I give instructions to recruit additional physicians from the hospital, put on the helmet and put on the climbing harness.

On the ride through the gorge, we see lifeless bodies drifting in the floodwaters deep down in the gorge. We fear the worst. After a few kilometers we reach the accident site: a broken guardrail, a steep rocky slope with bent trees and bushes and about 50 m in the depth a totally smashed tourist bus. It is located in the raging mountain stream, the seats free, the roof hangs sideways on a rock block. Some survivors have reached the road and are wandering aimlessly around, others are trying to climb the steep slope, but a larger number of people are lying deep down at the riverbank, partly lifeless, partly surrounded by survivors who are trying to tie them to the shore so that they are not swept away by the floods. In addition to the loud noise of the mountain stream, no sound can be heard. No crying, no moaning, desperate silence, shock.

I ask all those present not to leave the road, have fix ropes installed and mobilize mountain rescue, rescue personnel and doctors. I fix my rope to an EMS vehicle and abseil with the emergency medical kit to the accident site. There I see that the majority of the accident victims are children and adolescents. Numerous people had no signs of life. The bus is unreachable several meters from the riverbank in the raging flood. From the shore I can see some lifeless bodies between the seats. Meanwhile, the first mountain rescuers reach the scene and begin to abseil personnel and equipment. Now the recently established South Tyrolean emergency call center issues a disaster alarm throughout South Tyrol, which results in a chain of uncoordinated local alarms. Teams are set in motion from all directions, so that the narrow road can no longer hold the numerous vehicles. There are hardly any opportunities to turn around, so that an immense chaos arises during the transport of the injured, which hinders rescue efforts. In the air you can hear helicopters circling, but in the gorge there is no landing possibility and the use of the rescue winch directly at the accident site appears to be too risky due to the narrowness of the gorge. To make matters worse, due to the topography there is absolutely no radio or telephone contact with the outside world. The first reports, requests and instructions have to be given by couriers. There is neither an organized patient discharge area nor a treatment area.

At the riverbank, I try to triage roughly and have my firefighters lift the first severely injured onto the street where they are then taken over by the hospital doctors. We are able to reach the bus by ladder for the first time, which is dangerous during a flood. Together with 2 firefighters, I search the wreck, but most people no longer show any signs of life, only an older person lies deeply unconscious without any pain reaction in the middle aisle of the bus, has a pulse, a blood pressure of 80/40 mmHg and insufficient spontaneous respiration. After induction of anesthesia, intubation and ventilation, we bring the woman ashore, lift her onto the street where she suffers a cardiac arrest and dies after a resuscitation attempt. I go down to the river again, search the shore once more and find, strangely enough, a 12-year-old girl, deeply unconscious, pale and shallowly breathing, a few meters upstream. Meanwhile, the rescue chain is working better and the child is placed on a stretcher and brought up by pulley. An anesthesiologist and I try to do everything humanly possible to save the girl. We intubate, give oxygen, volume and vasopressors. We are able to stabilize the child and transport her by ambulance to the helicopter landing site, from where she is flown to the hospital. Unfortunately, this victim does not survive the accident either, but dies a few hours later from a rupture of the inferior vena cava.

Discussion
In total, 18 members of a tour group died in this accident. 20 people survived, some of them seriously injured. Taking into account the difficult topography of the accident site, the inadequate logistical preparation and the complete lack of disaster management, the emergency medical care was carried out without coordination, but so improvised that after about an hour all the seriously and moderately injured were rescued, treated and on their way to a hospital. The entire operation was made more difficult by the fact that EMS helicopters could not reach the accident site directly in the gorge and had to fly to a landing site that was approximately 5 km (3 miles) away at a valley mouth. From there, the seriously injured had to be brought to the ambulance first before they could be flown out.

In South Tyrol, the serious accident was like an earthquake that shook the responsible persons awake. On the one hand, it became clear at once how dangerous the journey was to one of the largest and best-known holiday regions in the world. The international press was full of negative headlines: "catastrophic road conditions, risky access to one of the most famous ski resorts in Europe". This alarmed the tourism industry and the demand for remediation was taken up. In the following years, the entire stretch of road was re-designed and a completely new route was laid out, mostly in tunnels. Today this stretch of road is one of the safest in the country and a crash into the gorge is virtually excluded.

On the other hand, there was a heated debate about the emergency medical care in South Tyrol after the accident; this had been neglected for years. No politician had reacted to the numerous night-time accidents, drink-driving was a misdemeanor and a mountain accident was a self-inflicted fate. Only one year before the accident, state law had ordered the establishment of control centers in all provinces; one year later, around-the-clock emergency services were set up in all hospitals throughout the country and now, for the first time, medically equipped physician-manned ambulances were deployed to emergencies.

18.1 Conclusion

It is a question of statistical frequency and geography when the next disaster relief operation will take place in a densely populated country [1]. In the case described here, we were absolutely not prepared for it. The example shows us how important it is to invest in safety and emergency medical care in a forward-looking manner. Whether we are today prepared for a mass influx of injured people of every size is still doubtful. The public is not used to acting, but often only reacts when something has gone wrong. The term prevention has its place in medicine, but less often in political bodies. Laws are still often formulated only when it is too late.

Reference

1. Ciottone G (2006) Disaster medicine, 1st ed. Elsevier-Mosby, Philadelphia

Shortness of Breath in Nursing Home

19

Luise Schnitzer

▶ This case shows very impressively how difficult—for all those involved—the handling of the topic of advance directives and their implementation can be. Often there are discrepancies between what is desired and what is wanted.

Our alarm keyword is "shortness of breath". We are already urgently expected by the nurse in the nursing home—she seems a little hectic and upset and leads us to a 96-year-old patient who is breathing heavily in bed. She has her eyes closed, is cyanotic and does not react to address. We first provide the patient with oxygen, which quickly brings her some relief, and now I try to find out something about the course of the disease from the patient. The nurse reports that the family doctor had already prescribed an antibiotic therapy a week ago, but this did not change the condition of the patient—on the contrary, it has now become worse and that is why she alarmed us. She can no longer guarantee the care of the patient in the nursing home and therefore asks us for hospitalization. The daughter of the patient, who has been following the report in silence so far, now interjects, clearly upset, with a trembling voice. It is clear that she is having a hard time controlling her emotions. She reports that her mother was admitted to the hospital several times in the last 3 months. After 1 week to 10 days she was discharged back to the nursing home, only to be readmitted to the hospital a few days later. She suffers from severe biventricular heart failure, renal failure and, due to a case of pronounced obesity, from massive congestion, edema on both legs and weeping ulcers on both lower legs. Already at her admission to the nursing home 2 years ago, an advance directive was created in which it was stipulated that the patient does not want to be treated on an intensive care unit anymore, that she does not want to be

L. Schnitzer (✉)
Charité University Medicine Berlin, Campus Benjamin Franklin,
Department of Cardiology and Pulmology, Berlin, Germany

V. Wenzel (ed.), *Case Studies in Emergency Medicine*,
https://doi.org/10.1007/978-3-662-67249-5_19

artificially ventilated or artificially fed and that she rejects any further treatment in a state that offers no more hope. She had also expressed the wish to die more frequently in recent weeks.

Only at my request does the nurse fetch the advance directive and now I am really surprised that we were even called. The nurse insists on hospitalization against the patient's wishes and against the daughter's wishes, because she does not want the patient to suffer and "they always helped her quite well in the hospital". She always came back in a better condition. In the meantime we have stopped the oxygen supply, the patient continues to breathe calmly, the skin color remains slightly livid. The nurse turns away indignantly and leaves the room. I talk to the daughter, tell her that I respect the patient's wish and that I will not take her to the hospital anymore. Since the patient is obviously not in pain, no medication is required. The daughter wants to stay with her mother and accompany her in the dying process. We leave the patient's room.

Out in the corridor, I meet the indignant nurse and try to calm her down. I ask her why she can't accept the patient's wish. I explain to her that we can't really help the patient anymore because at this point, there is no cure possible. She vehemently disagrees. "Medicine certainly has possibilities," she says, and now that the patient is no longer able to grasp the situation and can no longer speak for herself, she feels obliged as a nurse to act as her advocate. She argues that during her time on the intensive care unit she had already experienced apparently hopeless cases that had then recovered well and the same could be the case with this patient. I have many questions I'd like to ask her, that I ultimately keep to myself, because I can't expect any insight from the young woman, and so I leave the nursing home agitated. Although I don't question my decision, the unsatisfactory feeling remains that I haven't ended the mission optimally, because I failed to give the nurse an insight into my decision. I had the impression that the nurse "wanted to do something good" for the patient. On the other hand, it could not be excluded as a possibility that they wanted to "get rid of" a dying patient or that the nurse was overwhelmed with the process of dying. The patient died that same night; I did not have further communication with the nurse.

Discussion
The young nurse's unshakeable faith and the apparent trust in medical possibilities have confused and frustrated me. Doctors can heal, that is correct, and extend life spans, but we can often unnecessarily prolong the course of illness and suffering just as well [1–4]. It is no coincidence that the term "chronic critical illness" has developed, because certain illnesses can be treated but the patient can no longer be rehabilitated into a self-determined state [5]. These patients, for example, can be transferred from an intensive care unit to a ward, but often have to be readmitted to the intensive care unit quickly due to an acute deterioration. This "back and forth" between hospital and nursing home also existed in this patient and is inhuman, but usually continues as long as no one makes a decision. The boundaries of when we

overshoot the mark and do too much good are fluid and often creep in unnoticed [6, 7].

As doctors, we have the responsibility to ensure the welfare ("beneficence") of the human being, complying with the ban on causing harm ("Primum non nocere") and respecting the patient's right to self-determination (principle of autonomy). The principle of avoiding harm ("nonmaleficence") requires us to refrain from harmful interventions. It is also necessary to take into account fairness ("justice"), i.e. to use scarce resources sensibly and targeted. With the many developments in medicine and the enormous possibilities at our disposal, doctors are increasingly faced with ethical challenges. Do we have to treat every patient—administer every antibiotic therapy, carry out every dialysis, implant every pacemaker, carry out every heart catheterization [8]? Who decides on the welfare of the patient if he is no longer able to do so himself? I often experience the situation that patients are represented by an advocate who neither knows the patient nor has sufficient knowledge of his condition—but has to decide in a critical situation whether to withhold or carry out treatment. In the vast majority of cases I have experienced so far, the (legally appointed) representative has decided in favor of further treatment in order to be legally protected—and not always unjustifiably, as can be read in the press [9].

19.1 Conclusion

How far does the principle of non-harm ("Primum non nocere") have to be adhered to—when do therapies or omissions do "damage" to the patient? I think the duty to inform plays a very important role. To show the patient and the relatives the limits, to address the likely end and to discuss appropriate options, is essential. That this can be successful is shown in the admission to a hospice. Here dying is not taboo, death is expected and is a normal process. The fears may be expressed, understood and thus leave room for a dignified farewell. Such an open offer of conversation about the expected course of the disease, about the wishes of the patients should be required for all seriously chronically ill patients. Only the possibility to talk about it, eases the decision for the patient (and the relatives) in regards to how far the treatment should be advanced or not. In the hospital it is often observed that outside of normal working hours intensive care units are asked to take over patients who are in the process of dying when viewed more closely. Rarely, there is a "do-not-resuscitate" order, although there was enough time to discuss this with the patient. The cause is often a denial of death by the medical staff, the patient and the relatives or the inability to accept death. By continuing therapy regardless, new hopes are raised in patients and relatives, which are by no means justified. It seems unworthy to me to senselessly hurry a dying patient; each of us certainly imagines a dignified death differently. This should always be in the minds of medical staff: the dying process is part of our lives. With such a conversation the relatives, who usually do not have sufficient knowledge of medical basics, can also take away the fear of omitting something or feeling guilty.

References

1. Girshovich J (2014) Wem gehört der Tod? Vom Recht auf Leben und Sterbehilfe. Kein & Aber, Zürich. ISBN 978-3-0369-5648-0
2. Bayertz K, Frewer A (2002) Ethische Kontroversen am Ende des menschlichen Lebens. Palm & Enke, Erlangen. ISBN 3-7896-0584-0
3. Barmeyer J (2003) Praktische Medizinethik: die moderne Medizin im Spannungsfeld zwischen naturwissenschaftlichem Denken und humanitärem Auftrag – ein Leitfaden für Studenten und Ärzte, 2. stark überarb. Aufl. LIT-Verl., Münster, S 175. ISBN 3-8258-4984-8
4. Coors M, Grützmann T, Peters T (Hrsg) (2014) Interkulturalität und Ethik. Der Umgang mit Fremdheit in Medizin und Pflege, Edition Ethik Band 13, Edition Ruprecht, Göttingen. ISBN 978-3-8469-0162-5
5. Janssens U et al (2013) Therapiezieländerung und Therapiebegleitung in der Intensivmedizin – Deutsche interdisziplinäre Vereinigung für Intensiv- und Notfallmedizin. Med Klin Intensivmed Notfmed 108:47–52
6. Trzeczak S (2013) Notfallmedizin: Ethische Kompetenz und praktische Erfahrung. Dtsch Ärztebl 110:A706
7. Trzeczak S (2014) The medical–ethical dilemma regarding resuscitation decisions in emergency patients. Notf Rettungsmed 17:613–619
8. Bathe J (2012) Notarzteinsätze in Alten- und Pflegeheimen – der physician-manned ambulance als Lückenbüßer. Dissertation, Medizinische Fakultät Charité – Universitätsmedizin Berlin
9. Applebaum GE, King JE, Finucane TE (1990) The outcome of CPR initated in nursing homes. J Am Geriatr Soc 37:197–200

A Black Day for the EMS

Martin Messelken

▶ How much can an emergency physician really experience and carry in one day? In this case it becomes clear that a series of serious emergencies is possible on one day and represents an enormous challenge, which also has to be processed by the present helping persons, in order not to suffer any psychologically long-term trauma: even emergency physicians may ask for help.

It is election Sunday in the 1990s; the incumbent is re-elected. In a house attached to an authority, the family of the caretaker lives, who also works as a police officer at the authority. He should have helped already in the polling station; since his apartment door remains locked on several rings, it is forced open at noon. Due to the dramatic first impressions, an ambulance is alerted at 2:00 p.m. 7 min later, the following scene presents itself to the emergency physician and his EMS team: In the large attic apartment a breathtaking silence prevails, the first look falls on a huge Märklin model railway. Then 4 children are found dead in different rooms, they are between 8 and 15 years old. All lie face down in their beds and have gunshot wounds to the head and neck. No defensive struggle seems to have taken place anywhere, bloodstains that have already dried up can be seen. In the bedroom of the parents, the dead husband is found in a semi-sitting position with a pistol in his hand, he probably killed himself with a shot to the head. Next to him sits his motionless wife, she seems to be alive, although without any sensomotor reaction to the now people present. The gunshot wound she sustained is in the area of the left eye socket, where the blood that has flowed out there has already dried up. She remains unresponsive and does not speak a word, but has normal vital functions. Feedback is given to the EMS control center with the information that

M. Messelken (✉)
Bad Boll, Germany
e-mail: m.messelken@gmail.com

V. Wenzel (ed.), *Case Studies in Emergency Medicine*,
https://doi.org/10.1007/978-3-662-67249-5_20

only one patient is expected in the pre-alerted hospital. After rapid initial treatment, the approximately 50-year-old obese patient is transported by the ambulance to the emergency room of the responsible hospital of maximum care; from there she is later transferred to a neurosurgical hospital. Afterwards, the ambulance team returns to the scene of the accident together with the officers of the criminal police to carry out the autopsy of the 5 shot persons. The police investigations later reveal that the police officer executed his family with the service weapon after coming home from the night shift. Why this was possible without further ado was never clarified.

For the ambulance team there is an immediate follow-up mission with the message "child lies under collapsed wall". During a celebration of a family with a migrant background, children play on a fragile wall, which collapses and buries one of the children. The adults have already freed the lifeless 5-year-old child before the ambulance arrives. Cardiopulmonary resuscitation is started immediately, which is discontinued after 30 min without ever having at least temporarily established a spontaneous circulation. The present large family accompanies the treatment with loud sympathy, which of course does not leave the ambulance team and the emergency physician unaffected. Because of the obviously not natural cause of death, the police have to investigate here as well.

Shortly after midnight, another emergency call is required on a country road between 2 towns, as a pedestrian has been hit by a car. After arriving at the scene, the emergency physician can only determine the death with injuries that are incompatible with life. Since the accident originator has fled the scene, all that remains to be done is the documentation of death and a physical examination; here, too, the police investigates.

Discussion

If firearms are in a household, of course there is the danger that they will also be used in critical situations. Not only for the most justifiable self-defense, but also in situations of desperation and self-abandonment [1]. Family dramas occur again and again in such constellations. Apart from the fact that in the cases described here only one human life could be saved by emergency measures, the EMS and the emergency medical team had to cope with a considerable psychological stress situation. At that time in the 1990s, emergency chaplains or similar professional help such as crisis intervention teams were not or not everywhere available. Doctors, paramedics and police had to deal with such stressful situations more or less alone. This was done in different ways and depended more on the degree of socialization than on the need. Today there are excellent approaches for the prevention and avoidance of psychological stress in emergency and emergency medical services. Interestingly, the psychological help for emergency patients also plays a major role, because the more professional the dealing with the affected persons, the lower the stress for the emergency services themselves.

The acceptance of psychological stress in the workplace has been given the appropriate high priority in corporate health management [2, 3].

In addition, the autopsy is of considerable importance in connection with non-natural causes of death such as crime or accidental death. The emergency physician should document patient and environmental findings as well as pre-mortal treatment sufficiently and rather leave the determination of the time of death to forensic medicine [4]. Under no circumstances should one be tempted to certify a natural death if there is even the slightest hint of a possible opposite. Especially in connection with the death of older people, individual police officers tend to want to "close the files quickly".

20.1   Conclusion

Emergency Physicians and EMS staff must also be well equipped for high psychological stress, such as multiple child fatalities, even though the proportion of fatalities amounts to only about 3–5% of all emergency calls. In addition to a professional application of forensic principles and compliance with the applicable burial laws, an event-oriented psychosocial follow-up should take place not only in designated cases, but also in everyday life. EMS staff and emergency physicians may also ask for help.

References

1. Wintemute GJ (2008) Guns, fear, the constitution, and the public's health. N Engl J Med 358(14):1421–1424
2. D'Amelio RAC, Falkai P, Pajonk FG (2006)Psychological concepts and primary crisis intervention in emergency care Notfall & Rettungsmedizin. 9:194–204
3. Steil M (2010) Einsatzstress? So helfen Sie sich und anderen. ecomed SICHERHEIT, Landsberg am Lech
4. Nowak R (2013) Medikolegale Grundlagen. In: Dirks B (Hrsg) Die Notfallmedizin. Springer, Berlin, S 589–593

The Four Development Phases of a Medical Doctor

21

Joachim Koppenberg

▶ Which development phases does a medical doctor go through after his training in practice? And how can he deal with it if he is still in one of the first phases while facing a difficult medical problem? This case shows very clearly that even doctors should be aware of their humanity and fallibility in order to make their decisions with the necessary self-reflection.

The usual development states of a medical doctor after graduation can roughly be divided into four phases, which can certainly also have relevance for the type of treatment and the result of our patients. After graduation, one usually begins with the phase of "justified uncertainty" (1), which usually leads to the phase of "unjustified certainty" (2) after a few years and near the end of specialty training. After experiencing one or the other near-disaster or even real catastrophe in this phase, most people (apart from a few hard-boiled ones) slip into the phase of "unjustified uncertainty" (3). Only when one is then enlightened that, in addition to all the specialist knowledge and technical skills, one must also take into account other things between heaven and earth when making decisions, does one hopefully reach the phase of "justified certainty" (4) at some point, knowing full well that there will never be 100% certainty.

I am happy to report from my personal "Phase 2": After a strenuous routine operating day in cardiac anesthesia, I am suddenly called upon to fill in for a sick colleague for the city's physician-manned ambulance night shift in the same hospital. On the one hand, I owe the colleague a swapped shift, on the other hand I have just passed the specialist examination with flying colours and: Whoever

J. Koppenberg (✉)
Department of Anesthesiology, Pain Therapy and Emergency Medicine,
OSPIDAL – Center da sandà Engiadina Bassa, Scuol, Switzerland
e-mail: Joachim.Koppenberg@cseb.ch

V. Wenzel (ed.), *Case Studies in Emergency Medicine*,
https://doi.org/10.1007/978-3-662-67249-5_21

treats seriously ill and highly complex patients in cardiac anesthesia during the day will probably also be able to adequately care for a pre-hospital, urban emergency patient at night! So I am not particularly excited when, after 3 h of sleep, the call "asthma attack" wakes me up at 2 o'clock. After about 7 min drive, I enter the rather untidy-looking apartment of the 57-year-old patient, who is sitting at the kitchen table gasping for air. She looks very agitated, holding an asthma spray (fenoterol) in her right hand. While taking the first medical history, a 12-channel ECG (sinus rhythm, heart rate 138/min, no indications of a STEMI) and a pulse oximeter ($SpO_2 = 97\%$) are attached, and the blood pressure is measured (RR $= 180/100$ mmHg). Due to the severe shortness of breath, the patient can only give "snippets" of information and confirms the reported symptoms of "asthma attack" in the case of a long-standing asthma condition (basic medication with inhaled corticosteroid, long-acting $ß_2$ agonist and oral theophylline). While taking the medical history, 4 l/min oxygen is applied via a nasal cannula.

According to the patient, she went to bed at around 11 pm and then woke up spontaneously at midnight due to increasing shortness of breath. This may be rather unusual, but asthma attacks usually come quite irregularly and are not predictable. Therefore, she took another dose of oral theophylline, as she could usually "adjust herself quite well". In addition, she has inhaled the short-acting $ß_2$-mimetic (fenoterol) several times since then, but the attack has become worse despite this. In addition, a still ongoing history of nicotine abuse of 70 pack years can be determined, which must suffice for me as a non-smoker as "receipt" for the current attack. Lung auscultation reveals a weakened breath sound on both sides, but without signs of spasticity or humming or whistling. A beginner would probably have been suspicious here—but of course I interpret this in the context of the severe asthma attack as "silent lung"—quite professional! After the patient has practically administered all asthma medications herself, I insert an i.v. access and consider what other treatment options are left for such a severe asthma attack (prednisolone? Terbutaline s.c.? Reproterol i.v.? Intubation with ketamine?). In the meantime, I also inquire about allergies (none) and other comorbidities (poorly controlled hypertension—as measured—and hypercholesterolemia). The patient mentions left thoracic pain in conversation, which she attributes to forced respiration. For the first time, I become alert during this intervention and ask for more details. The pain is continuous, not related to respiration, and cannot be influenced by palpation. The pain has increased steadily since the beginning of the "asthma attack" and is currently rated at 6/10 on the Verbal Rating Scale. In addition, this has a burning character, but no radiation is denied. A repeat blood pressure measurement still shows values of 190/100 mmHg. For the first time, I leave my nightly "autopilot mode" and go through possible differential diagnoses: Of course, it could also be an acute coronary syndrome or a pulmonary embolism. So what's next? Maybe this is even more likely—isn't the room air saturation at 97%? Why only now do I notice that this does not fit a severe asthma attack at all! Now I consider the intersection of the further therapy options, which can be justified by both diagnoses. First of all, it would certainly not be a bad idea to lower the blood pressure. After two doses of nitro sublingual, the blood pressure decreases to 148/90 mmHg and the patient reports at the same time a slight improvement in pain and shortness of breath—an asthma attack does not usually respond to nitro spray! Thereafter, I fractionate (2 mg each) morphine i.v. to the patient for analgesia until an improvement in symptoms on the Verbal Rating Scale from 6 to 2. At the same time, a nitroperfusor is installed, as I want to forego the injection of a beta blocker and aspirin due to the known asthma history.

While on the one hand the actual problem of the patient (acute coronary syndrome) is becoming increasingly clear to me, on the other hand I am getting more and more angry about my own blindness and ignorance so far. In parallel, the transport to the emergency room is prepared and carried out with the suspicion of an acute coronary syndrome. There laborchemically a Non-STEMI-myocardial infarction is confirmed, which is treated immediately by means of a percutaneous coronary intervention.

Discussion

What had happened? Now first of all quite simply—the patient initially had a nocturnal ischemic cardiac event, the symptoms of which she associated with her long-standing asthma and therefore also treated accordingly—with β-mimetics (fenoterol) and caffeine-like (theophylline) drugs, which increasingly worsened the ischemia—these drugs are not without reason in an acute coronary syndrome contraindicated! And the worse the patient felt, the more of these drugs she used—a real iatrogenic and exogenous vicious circle! But why hadn't I seen this mechanism before, let myself be deceived for so long and, despite my current work in cardiac anesthesia, not immediately recognized or at least considered the acute coronary syndrome? Also quite simply—because it is human! In fact, we physicians are only too human and are all too easily caught up in typical cognitive mistakes. The reason for this is based in the so-called heuristic. Here, informal or fuzzy rules are created from experience values, which in complex situations leads to taking cognitive shortcuts and thus finding quick and pragmatic solutions with limited knowledge under time pressure [1, 2]. This does indeed often lead to adequate solutions, but unfortunately these heuristics can simply and fundamentally be wrong. We want to take a closer look at some typical pitfalls in the case described.

First of all, it all starts with the inner attitude, which I typically took on in phase 2 ("unjustified security"). Self-confident and convinced that I was experienced and saddle-fast, this did not exactly promote critical self-reflection, which is always required in the medical profession. First, the clinical picture "asthma attack" was confirmed by the situation on site and the patient herself. Here I first fell into the "availability error" trap ("availability bias"), which describes the tendency to take the cognitively "most available" option—the most obvious one—[4]. This was practically parallel to the "anchoring bias", one of the common cognitive pitfalls. This states that the first impression gained has a disproportionate influence on further thinking behavior and that one is reluctant to deviate from the first offered hypothesis. This goes so far that contradictory information is ignored—as in this case a completely normal room air oxygen saturation of 97% in an allegedly severe asthma attack. On the contrary, the so-called "confirmation bias" was committed: Here, hints are sought and perceived, which confirm one's own working diagnosis—in this case the bland pulmonary auscultation finding, which I reinterpreted as part of my working diagnosis "asthma attack" to a "silent lung" in order to not have to call my working hypothesis into question. Only a symptom that was no longer appropriate at all (chest pain) had torn me out of my self-confidence and, in the truest sense of the word, "awakened" me and made me think and search for possible differential diagnoses.

21.1 Conclusion

The most important lesson I learned from this case was that, in addition to the purely technical knowledge and skills, there are other skills needed for optimal patient care, which I had not heard or learned about during my studies and my previous medical training. What is really fatal is that these heuristic errors influence our medical thinking on a daily basis and thus have a decisive influence on the outcome of our patients. Although it is of course extremely difficult not to be led astray by these heuristics, which we have trained ourselves in all our lives, it is worth taking a closer look at these modes of thinking and error models. The sharpest weapon we have against these mental errors is "situational awareness". This describes the degree of agreement between our view and reality in certain situations, which we can only increase by constantly questioning the situation and our working hypothesis. One could also say quite banally: keep a cool head and an overview [3].

In order to finally reach phase 4 of "justified certainty", it is advisable to follow the saying that has been hanging on my locker door since then as a daily reminder: "Don't believe everything you think!"

References

1. Gausmann P, Henninger M, Koppenberg J (2022) Patient safety management, 2nd edition. De Gruyter, Berlin
2. St. Pierre M, Hofinger G (2014) Human Factors und Patientensicherheit in der Akutmedizin. Springer Verlag, Heidelberg
3. Dobelli R (2011) Die Kunst des klaren Denkens. Hanser, München
4. Wachter RM (2010) Fokus Patientensicherheit: Fehler vermeiden, Risiken managen. In: Koppenberg J, Gausmann P, Henninger M (Hrsg). ABW-Wissenschaftsverlag, Berlin

Fall into Garden Pond

Luise Schnitzer

▶ Interventions in which the patients are very small are always very emotional for all involved and can also be quite stressful in terms of debriefing. This case picks up on such a situation and also addresses the developments that have changed over time.

2-year-old twins fall into a garden pond. After a maximum of 10 min, during which the children are unsupervised, the older brother finds the two lifeless and alarms the father, who rescues the children from the water and then immediately alarms the fire department. When I arrive, I find two lifeless children who are clearly hypothermic. The ECG shows asystole, the pupils are maximally dilated in both children and do not react to light. The members of the fire department are committed to performing chest compressions on both children—my rescue assistants are working with high pressure—I intubate the boy first, then the girl, place an intravenous access one after the other in both and inject epinephrine. In both cases, a sinus rhythm appears after a short time, but only with a frequency of 80/min and they remain pulseless, the pupils remain maximally dilated. In the meantime, reinforcement has arrived—a physician colleague takes over the resuscitation attempt of the boy and I continue to take care of the girl. Both receive epinephrine again and are constantly treated with chest compressions and ventilated—interrupted again and again by suctioning the large volume of water that the children have aspirated.

After about 15 min of cardiopulmonary resuscitation, we can feel a pulse, but the heart rate remains insufficient at about 80/min, so the chest compressions are

L. Schnitzer (✉)
Charité University Medicine Berlin, Campus Benjamin Franklin,
Department of Cardiology and Pulmology, Berlin, Germany
e-mail: l.schnitzer@gmx.de; l.schnitzer@gmx.de

V. Wenzel (ed.), *Case Studies in Emergency Medicine*,
https://doi.org/10.1007/978-3-662-67249-5_22

continued. In the meantime, many professional responders have arrived—even the press has gathered. I have never experienced such focused and harmonious cooperation between professional responders and the fire department: the media representatives are shielded, the stretchers are prepared, the rescuers who perform chest compressions are swapped out seamlessly, new oxygen bottles appear before they are actually needed. Since both children are clearly hypothermic, we decide to transport them while performing chest compressions and take them to two different hospitals. After my handover, I receive skeptical looks, but the hospital colleagues resuscitate with commitment for another 2 h—the girl is even being resuscitated for a total of 3 long hours—until the circulation is stable and the heart rate is sufficient. The core temperature of the girl upon admission is <28 °C (<82.4 °F) and is kept at 32–34 °C (89.6-93.2 °F) and is only slowly raised in the course of time, so that she only has a normal temperature 72 h after admission to the hospital. After an initially encouraging course in her and stable respiratory function, oxygenation deteriorates dramatically: in the CT, increasing bilateral pulmonary infiltrates are detected, a sepsis with multi-organ failure develops and finally the girl is treated with high-frequency oscillation ventilation. On the 7th day we can breathe a sigh of relief; the respiratory and organ functions improve and sedation can be reduced. She recovers surprisingly quickly and can be transferred to a ward on the 11th day healthy and without neurological damage.

The procedure proves just as dramatic at the other hospital—the boy has been resuscitated for another 1½ h, his core temperature is <27 °C (<80.6 °F) upon admission, the pupils remain dilated and do not react to light. The only significant difference to the current course of his sister's illness is that he has a seizure, which also occurs occasionally afterwards. His intensive care course is much simpler than his sister's; the temperature is quickly raised to 37 °C (98.6 °F). He is ventilated without complications, circulation is supported mildly with catecholamines as with his sister. He can be extubated after 6 days. The dramatic thing is that after sedation is stopped, the boy is diagnosed with a severe neurological deficit syndrome with spasticity and muscle spasms.

This event has affected all those involved deeply. I was told by a firefighter who was involved that he no longer felt able to continue on duty. He was transferred to the rescue control center so that he would no longer be affected by the direct course of events. The family writes me a small update every year, reports on the well-being and progress of the children. They invite me and my paramedic from the physician-manned ambulance to visit them, which we are happy to do. Deeply impressed by the selfless and loving care of the parents, we can experience a lively 5-year-old little girl who likes to go to kindergarten and loves her brother very much. The boy suffers from spasticity, looks very awake and curious, but can only formulate incomprehensible words for us. Approximately 16 years later, I receive an invitation to a lecture that the two "children"—now young adults—are to give to a professional audience; the topic of their talk is: Communication with each other—how we communicate. It is an honor for me to attend this lecture. I sit in awe in the auditorium and experience how the sister introduces and comments on the small lecture and the boy tells us about his hobbies using technical means, how he practiced early on with picture boards with his mother and later with his father how he was trained in using computers. The young man is able to express his thoughts and feelings; he can express his anger, for example, that people do not let him finish. He types his sentences into a computer, which does take some time, and a speech computer then translates his texts into speech for those around him. I wish for myself and for everyone else, to muster that little bit of patience to listen—because he and others like him certainly have a lot to say.

Discussion

The children have been treated differently—therapeutic hypothermia was maintained in the girl, in the boy this was not carried out; it is possible that this made a difference in neurological recovery. However, we do not know anything specific about the time of the accident in the two children. It is possible that there were actually time differences in the time of hypoxia that were decisive. The girl had a complicated course with severe sepsis and multiple organ failure [1], possibly due to hypothermia. The development and improvement of therapeutic hypothermia protects or reduces neurological damage [2, 3] and is now standard in the post-treatment of cardiopulmonary resuscitated patients [2–4]. It is conceivable that the differences in rewarming explained the different course. The guidelines for cardiopulmonary resuscitation recommend a rewarming after therapeutic hypothermia in an order of magnitude of $\leq 0.5\,°C$ ($32.9\,°F$)/hour, a limit that (of course under other conditions) was probably adhered to by the girl, but not by the boy. However, a faster rewarming using a heart-lung machine or extracorporeal membrane oxygenation in severe hypothermia, for example after an avalanche accident, is also discussed [5]. The boy recovered quite well after the initial severe neurological concerns. The tireless care of the parents and siblings certainly played a decisive role.

Another aspect is the post-traumatic stress of this deployment in the professional rescuers. Resuscitating two small children is a special challenge for everyone involved, not only in the technical process, but also in processing what has happened. "It could have been my child!" was surely a thought on everyone's mind involved; but also: "Did I do everything right?", "Did I miss something?", "Was it my fault?" These questions haunt you and have to be processed. Fortunately, today there is the possibility—much more so than before—to cope better with such traumatic events through conversations with trained personnel from crisis intervention teams and not to repress them.

22.1 Conclusion

In addition to the assumption that unexpectedly excellent results happen again and again, it is always difficult to classify and assess neurological findings, especially in children, in a long-term perspective. Today we are additionally able to develop hidden talents and compensate for disabilities with technical aids. Only a decade earlier, the boy would probably not have found a way to communicate with the outside world and would have been limited to familiar domestic life. Today he has the opportunity to communicate with everyone and to learn a profession according to his personal abilities.

References

1. Vargas Hein O, Tritsch A, von Buch C, Kox WJ, Spies C (2004) Mild hypothermia after near drowning in twin toddlers. Crit Care 8:R353–357
2. Rittenberger JC, Callaway CW (2013) Temperature management and modern post-cardiac arrest care. N Engl J Med 369:2262–2263
3. Peberdy MA, Callaway CW, Neumar RW et al (2010) Post-cardiac arrest care: 2010 American Heart Association guidelines for cardiopulmonary resuciation and emergency cardiovascular care. Circulation 122(Suppl 3):S768–786 (Errata, Circulation 2011; 123(6):e237, 124(15):e403
4. Palmers PJ, Hiltrop N, Ameloot K, Timmermans P, Derdinande B, Sinnaeve P, Nieuwendijk R, Malbrain ML (2014) From therapeutic hypothermia towards targeted temperature management: a decade of evolution. Anaesthesiol Intensive Ther 47(2):156–161
5. Mair P, Brugger H, Mair B, Moroder L, Ruttmann E (2014) Is extracorporeal rewarming indicated in avalanche victims with unwitnessed hypothermic cardiorespiratory arrest? High Alt Med Biol 15(4):500–503. https://doi.org/10.1089/ham.2014.1066

Two Pathologies

23

Hans-Richard Arntz

▶ Not always, as this case shows, are the symptoms clearly attributable to a disease picture and not always is only one disease picture present—but fortunately, as in this situation, there is a therapy that can treat two pathologies at the same time.

We are alarmed with the keyword "sudden unconsciousness" on a summer day early in the evening and, after a short flight with the EMS helicopter, arrive at the patient's house about 15 min after the event. A 58-year-old patient—as we learn from the physician at the scene of the accident—collapsed after a car journey of about 6 h, interrupted only by short breaks, and was unable to get up again. The past medical history reveals a slight hypertension and occasional migraine attacks. Both have been completely stable for a long time with beta-blocker therapy, according to the patient. We see a conscious, pain-free patient who is oriented in time and space, but not in terms of her symptoms. There is an obviously acute complete hemiparesis on the left and an indicated dysarthria. The patient reports that during the car journey in the last few hours she noticed twice short-term visual disturbances in the form of a flicker scotoma in the right visual field and a tingling sensation on the right side of the tongue. Both are known to her as prodromal symptoms in the event of an impending migraine attack. After several attempts at explanation, the patient finally agrees to be transported by our EMS helicopter to a neurological center for immediate cranial computed tomography. The multiple explanation attempts are necessary because the patient categorically denies the diagnosis of a stroke with hemiplegia in the context of an apoplexy-related acute neglect syndrome. We don't want to lose a minute because of the

H.-R. Arntz (✉)
Charité, University Medicine Berlin, Campus Benjamin Franklin,
Department of Cardiology and Pulmology, Berlin, Germany
e-mail: HRArntz@t-online.de

V. Wenzel (ed.), *Case Studies in Emergency Medicine*,
https://doi.org/10.1007/978-3-662-67249-5_23

option of thrombolytic therapy. During the entire pre-hospital treatment, including the helicopter transport, the patient remains completely stable and pain-free. However, the neglect seems to be lost when the patient is unloaded from the helicopter, because for the first time she anxiously asks whether she really has a stroke.

Immediately upon being handed over to the neurologists who had been alerted in advance and were already waiting—no longer under continuous monitoring at this point—the patient apparently has a seizure. However, the atypical pallor that sets in after a few seconds and the subsequent cessation of breathing shortly thereafter prove that it is an Adam-Stokes attack. In this case, the cause is an acute circulatory arrest due to fibrillation, as can be seen on a monitor set up quickly; immediate cardiopulmonary resuscitation was initiated. After a few minutes and one defibrillation, circulation is stable and detectable again, but intubation and ventilation as well as short-term sedation are necessary. The ECG registered at this point shows the signs of an acute inferior myocardial infarction with ST-segment elevations in II, III and aVF. Immediately afterwards, a cranial computed tomogram is performed, which, like a transcranial Doppler sonogram, turns out to be unimpressive. After a short discussion between cardiologists and neurologists, despite the limited ability to assess the neurological status, the decision is made to initiate systemic thrombolysis therapy and to forego coronary intervention for the time being. The 100-minute time window since the onset of the insult at this point gives hope for a good thrombolysis result. The possibilities of coronary intervention, on the other hand, seem secondary. In addition, the consideration that thrombolysis could also be an effective therapy for myocardial infarction, i.e. both diseases could be approached with the same therapeutic principle, plays a role. However, thrombolysis must be carried out with a reduced dose for myocardial infarction. In addition, because of the risk of massive intracranial bleeding, the usual adjuvant therapy with aspirin and heparin for myocardial infarction is not possible. Thrombolysis is initiated approximately 120 min after the onset of neurological symptoms with rt-PA (0.9 mg/kg, initial bolus 10% of the dose and administration of the remaining dose over 60 min). The patient wakes up spontaneously 2 h after the end of thrombolysis and is fully oriented after a short time. Clinically and neurologically, at this point there is only an internuclear ophthalmoplegia on the right and an incomplete vertical gaze palsy upwards. There is also a hemiataxia on the right and a slight hemiparesis on the left. All symptoms largely disappear within the next few days, with the exception of a hand-held disturbance of fine motor skills on the right.

In the EKG, Q-waves develop inferiorly as an expression of an ongoing acute posterior wall infarction. The CK rises to a maximum of 186 U/l and the CK-MB to 38 U/l; the Troponin-T rapid test is positive. There is hypokalemia at the time of ventricular fibrillation of 3.3 mmol/l. Clinical signs of heart failure do not develop. Rhythm disorders are also not observed. In a cerebral MRI performed 5 days after the event, multiple ischemic lesions are demarcated right pontine, left cerebellar and right fronto-parietal. In the following cardiological follow-up examinations, hypokinesia of the inferior wall of the left ventricle with discrete relative mitral insufficiency grade 0–1 is found in the ventriculography during cardiac catheterization. No significant coronary stenoses are detected. In the transesophageal echo, after contrast agent administration, contrast agent passage into the left atrium is seen as a sign of an open foramen ovale, which is prophylactically treated with an "occluder".

Discussion

This is the unusual case of successful simultaneous systemic thrombolysis treatment of brain and myocardial infarction as a result of the coincidence of these events; etiopathogenetically, 3 considerations can be made. Cerebral infarcts are very rare complications of migraine attacks; the incidence is about 1/100,000/year. Inflammatory changes in the vessels, embolisms and arterial dissections are discussed. Although the patient had experienced typical migraine symptoms for the first time in years on the trip, the documentation of multiple ischemic lesions is an important argument against the assumption of a migraine-associated brain infarction. It would also be unusual for a migraine-induced insult without anamnestic indications of a complicated migraine course (so-called migraine accompagnée). Patients with this course of disease experience transient neurological deficits, equivalent to an increased risk of ischemic stroke. The initial cardiac symptom-free course and ventricular fibrillation in the context of an acute myocardial infarction documented after ischemic insult also suggest that the infarction could have occurred secondary to the stroke-associated acute stress situation. However, the most likely cause is a paradoxical embolism. This is supported by the fact that the brain infarctions occurred in multiple locations with proven patent foramen ovale. Paradoxical brain embolisms as the cause of so-called "cryptogenic strokes" are predominantly observed in younger people under the age of 55 [1]. Our patient was at least not far outside this risk age with 58 years. Although very rare, a myocardial infarction caused by a paradoxical embolism is possible. The triggering of the events by several embolisms of very fresh "paradoxical" thrombi, e.g. from the leg vein area after prolonged sitting during the car ride, is also supported by the excellent thrombolysis effect.

23.1　Conclusion

The occluder prophylaxis used at the time for persistent foramen ovale is a procedure used today primarily for patients with contraindications for anticoagulation [2]. Prophylaxis with anticoagulation is preferred, for which, in addition to the classical therapy with vitamin K antagonists, several new drugs are now available [3].

References

1. Homma S, Sacco RL (2005) Patent foramen ovale and stroke. Circulation 112:1063–1072
2. Freixa X, Arzamendi D, Tzikas A, Noble S, Basmadjian A, Garceau P, Ibrahim R (2014) Cardiac procedures to prevent stroke: patent foramen ovale closure/left atrial appendage occlusion. Can J Cardiol 30:87–95
3. Gómez-Outes A, Terleira-Fernández AI, Calvo-Rojas G, Suárez-Gea ML, Vargas-Castrillón E (2013) Dabigatran, Rivaroxaban, or Apixaban versus Warfarin in patients with nonvalvular atrial fibrillation: a systematic review and metaanalysis of subgroups. Thrombosis 2013:640723. https://doi.org/10.1155/2013/640723

High-rise Building on Fire

24

Sven Wolf

> ▶ This case shows that every emergency physician can also find themselves in a situation where they have to make quick and competent decisions in order to save the lives of the people involved. Therefore, as is also very clear here, prevention begins in the head, namely before such a situation arises.

The alarm of the on-call senior emergency physician in the event of a mass casualty incident is received at 10:00 pm on a cold autumn day after feedback from the first arriving fire brigade in a high-rise settlement. On the 2nd floor of a 7-story residential building, an apartment is in full blaze with flames leaping to the 3rd floor. Both stairwells are completely smoked and drive many of the reported 58 residents to the upper floors on their balconies. A woman falls from the 3rd floor onto a lawn. The first arriving physician is met by numerous residents from both stairwells. There is a German-Russian language confusion, some residents cough loudly. Before several passers-by pull the physician by the sleeve to the rear of the building to the multiple traumatized "jumper", he orders 2 policemen to collect all residents on a nearby lawn. During intubation of the patient on the lawn, the physician hands over the scene to the on-call senior emergency physician. After ordering the immediate transport of the multiple trauma woman in the company of the physician to a hospital of maximum care, the senior emergency physician first needs 5 min to find his responsible organizational leader of the EMS. This turns out to be just as difficult as the subsequent joint reconnaissance, since the affected building complex can only be reached from 3 sides by footpath. In the area of the affected stairwells, the two policemen commissioned meanwhile intercept 15 residents from the house, but can only convince them with considerable

S. Wolf (✉)
Department of Emergency Medicine, DIAKOVERE Friederikenstift, Hannover, Germany
e-mail: drsvenwolf@web.de

V. Wenzel (ed.), *Case Studies in Emergency Medicine*,
https://doi.org/10.1007/978-3-662-67249-5_24

difficulty and language barriers to wait for the senior emergency physician on the area of the affected lawn; a quick assessment of the 15 residents is carried out under the usual local identification with red and white velcro. 2 elderly women on foot with coughing and dyspnea are handed over directly to two ambulance crews, the remaining residents are initially marked with "white". Meanwhile, 2 more ambulance crews arrive from different directions and report to the senior emergency physician about several "clusters" of suspected patients around the building complex. After consulting with the fire department's overall incident commander, the EMS organizational leader then determines a defined larger deployment area "EMS" in about 200 m / 650 feet distance to the fire object via the EMS control center, where an emergency response vehicle is being used as a reporting center. A team of paramedics and 2 volunteer firefighters are now "guarding" the patient drop-off area on the lawn, while the senior emergency physician, the organizational leader of emergency services, and a physician-manned ambulance team move in opposite directions around the building complex to explore and assess the situation. They communicate with each other using 2-meter radios. Both teams first requisition a man who speaks German and Russian from the patient gathering point as an interpreter. 2 factors make it very difficult for the teams to identify additional potential patients: first, about 300 relatives, friends, and onlookers are streaming out of the surrounding buildings to the scene of the incident; second, it is starting to rain heavily. The large emergency response vehicle from the fire department has now arrived in the easily visible deployment area "EMS". Due to the weather, both teams are now sending the patients they have seen directly to the large emergency response vehicle instead of to the patient gathering point on the lawn. The local rapid response team with its EMS station now arrives in the deployment area. The leader of the rapid response team estimates that it will take 45–60 min to completely set up the EMS station in the area of the incident. Despite all the difficulties, both assessment teams are able to identify and assess 22 more residents of the affected house by then. Almost all of them fall into assessment category III (slightly injured, postponed treatment priority). For this reason, the senior emergency physician is foregoing the complete set-up of the EMS station in favor of an inflatable quick response tent in the area of the deployment area and large emergency response vehicle. About 20 min after the departure of the two assessment teams, they meet again on the lawn in the entrance area at the original patient drop-off area. To their surprise, there is now only one of the two firefighters who were originally commissioned there. Upon inquiry, he reports that "someone" had come and informed them about the "dissolution of the assembly point". Before they knew it, the 13 patients under their supervision had disappeared in all directions. It is later not possible to reconstruct who this "someone" could have been among the 155 emergency personnel. Since the large emergency response vehicle also features a carbon monoxide-hemoglobin measurement, it is now being used as an assessment point for the re-evaluation of patients in the deployment area. In addition to the multiple trauma woman, this allows 24 more residents who may have been exposed to smoke to be assessed and categorized over the course of time (1 × assessment category I "red" acute vital threat =>

immediate treatment, $3 \times$ assessment category II "yellow" seriously injured/ill => postponed treatment urgency, $12 \times$ assessment category III "green" slightly injured/sick => later, if necessary, outpatient treatment). 8 people refuse transport, the remaining 17 are admitted to the hospital. Fortunately, retrospectively, no serious pulmonary complications occur among the non-assessed, or non-re-evaluated, "disappeared" patients/residents.

Discussion

In the following maneuver review, it was difficult to define clear errors or improvement suggestions from the complex course of the operation. Essentially, the first arriving paramedic and the senior emergency physician or the organizational leader of the EMS team did everything right. The difficult and unsatisfactory course of the operation ultimately resulted from a combination of several unfavorable factors, such as high and unclear number of potential patients, very confusing location, difficult order of the location, insufficient or missing cordon, language barriers, weather (night, rain) and a variety of different emergency services (regular EMS, rapid response team, fire department, police). Although a mass casualty incident situation is very rare and difficult to standardize, every paramedic should get used to the idea that he or she usually has to take over the complete range of tasks as senior emergency physician on the first arriving ambulance [1]! As a rule, there are no "arrival or rescue deadlines" defined for the on-call senior emergency physician so far, so that everything from 6 to 60 min is conceivable and possible according to experience. Unlike in the individual EMS, there are no comprehensive "guidelines" of the professional societies for the senior emergency physician, but only general, guiding "cornerstones" of action [2–4], which have to be adapted to the geographical and local EMS structure of each deployment area. The individual screening systems in the German-speaking area (e.g. mSTaRT [5]) are now adapted to the local conditions, well established and tried and tested [3]. Not only as on-call senior emergency physician, but also as on-call paramedic, one should know the local "system" (quick screening, labeling, patient attachment cards, rapid response teams infrastructure, etc.) with its strengths and weaknesses. The latter is best crystallized in regular exercises, war games and appropriate debriefings [4]. Regardless of the local conditions, there are a few "cornerstones" [1, 2, 4, 6], which keep reappearing for the (provisional) senior emergency physician: Never separate from your organizational leader EMS (or physician-manned ambulance driver), take a clear identification with corresponding (blue) vests, observe local command and communication structures (e.g. overall incident commander, lower incident sections, radio call names, etc.). The core tasks of the senior emergency physician consist in the quickest possible, structured screening, the core task of the organizational leader EMS in maintaining communication and documentation. The core tasks that leading paramedics and EMS organizational leaders have in common are the order of the location, coordination of medical or technical rescue, timely situation reports to the rescue control center as well as requisition of additional forces and expansion or withdrawal of the mass casualty incident level.

The space order is often underestimated and primarily left to the EMS control center, but it is later only very difficult to correct [7]. The potential provisional space "EMS" must be determined as quickly as possible, ideally already on the approach, using maps/local knowledge and communicated to the rescue control center [6]. While the determination of the deployment area for the rescue station can usually be done at a later time after arriving at the scene of the accident, the primary patient collection point (DIN 13050) must be determined immediately. Ideal are weather-protected, fixed premises such as large corridors, gymnasiums or courtyards. If only an outdoor area is available, this is to be marked as quickly as possible to avoid the disappearance of patients, "fenced in" and if possible shielded (flagging tape, gauze, fire safety lines, blankets, "wagon fortress" with vehicles, tents, etc.) [1, 2]. Pedestrian patients and those in need of help in their distress and panic often tend to run to the first recognizable rescue vehicle ("crystallization nucleus"). If there is no suitable patient support, the senior emergency physician can take advantage of this and, for example, position the first arriving ambulance in a well-visible defined approach point/collection point near the damage site.

While patients in sighting category I and sighting category II must be stabilized and transported as quickly as possible on site, patients in sighting category III should be screened, cared for and then re-evaluated near the scene of the accident. For example, in the event of predominantly "care situations", it may make sense not to set up the EMS station at all, but to use the personnel of the rapid response team situationally from the outset rather for care [7]. Appropriate tasks (-changes) must be delegated clearly and binding by the medical operation leader (senior emergency physician/EMS organizational leader EMS service/possibly consultant medical care) [1, 6].

24.1 Conclusion

Any physician could unintentionally find themselves in the role of (provisional) senior emergency physician. Unlike in the individual medicine of the regular EMS, there are usually only framework guidelines for the tasks of the senior emergency physician in the event of a mass casualty incident. These mainly concern operational principles such as screening, communication, documentation and order of the location. In addition to these basic principles, it will be a great help for the affected (potential) senior emergency physician if he (preferably together with his physician-manned ambulance driver/EMS organizational leader ambulance service) regularly informs himself about the local deployment structures in the event of a mass casualty incident and corresponding special features. Prevention starts here in the head [6]! Furthermore, it makes sense for the twosome to think through and discuss randomly invented deployment situations and scenarios "[(…) if there were an overturned bus there, where could we define patient drop-off, staging area, etc.? (…)]" or to simulate them with professional guidance in seminars [1, 8].

References

1. Pajonk FG, Dombroesky WR (2006) Panik bei Großschadensereignissen. Not Rettungsmed 9:280–286
2. Adams HA, Krettek C, Lange C, Unger C (Hrsg) (2013) Patientenversorgung im Großschadens- und Katastrophenfall: Medizinische und organisatorische Herausforderungen jenseits der Individualmedizin. Deutscher Ärzteverlag, Köln
3. Beck A, Bayeff-Filloff M, Kanz KG, Sauerland S, AG Notfallmedizin der DGU (2005) Algorithmus für den Massenanfall von Verletzten. Notf Rettungsmed 8:466–473
4. Schweigkofler U (2011) Katastrophenmedizin – ein etwas modifiziertes medizinisches Versorgungskonzept. Tagung: Katastrophen und Großereignisse bewältigen. BGU + IVM Frankfurt a. M.
5. Kanz KG, Hornburger P, Kay MV et al (2006) The mSTaRT algorithm for mass casualty incident management. Notf Rettungsmed 9:264–270
6. Dirks B (2006) Management of mass incidents by the chief emergency physician. Notf Rettungsmed 9:333–346
7. Beneker J, Marx F, Mieck F, Reinhold T, Ekkernkamp A (2014) Großunfälle – Erfahrungen aus drei Realeinsätzen. Notarzt 30:206–217
8. Roesberg H, Habers J, Oppermann S (2006) Simulation als Vorbereitung auf nicht alltägliche Rettungsdiensteinsätze. Rettungsdienst 29:32–34

Child with Head Injury

Martin Dünser

▶ There is nothing that does not exist—this statement becomes very clear in this case. A foreign country, poor treatment conditions and a special injury meet and present the treating doctors with a special challenge.

It is hot—as every day. It is turbulent on the intensive care unit of the hospital in Ifakara/Tanzania—as every day. Most patients treated here have an infection: respiratory infections paired with malaria, obstetric complications, preeclampsia and trauma are other common admission diagnoses. Children are usually admitted to the intensive care unit due to a malaria infection, a respiratory infection (±malaria), diarrhea with dehydration or burns. Today is surgery day. We expect 5 patients after open prostatectomy. The procedure only takes 15–20 min, but has a very high complication rate. In particular, the "transurethral resection of the prostate" (TURP) syndrome is very common due to postoperative bladder flushing. The preparations are interrupted when I am called to the operating suite in the other part of the hospital. Stay nice on the concrete sidewalks and don't shortcut over the grassy areas—there are snakes there.

In front of the operating room, a mother is sitting with an approximately 8-month-old child in her arms. The child is visibly scared. A wool cap hangs from his head. Next to him is the surgeon, who has been waiting for me and tells me the story: A collapsing fence with a protruding nail had hit the child on the head. In the process, the nail pierced the wool cap and then got stuck in the skull bone. The mother immediately removed the fence with the nail; but the wool cap remained stuck in the wound. There was never any loss of consciousness. The child is also

M. Dünser (✉)
Department of Anesthesiology and Critical Care Medicine, Kepler University Hospital, Linz, Austria
e-mail: Martin.Duenser@kepleruniklinikum.at

uneventful on a gross neurological level at the time of my examination. Therefore, a relevant injury to intracranial structures seems unlikely to me. The surgeon is concerned that the wool cap may have been displaced into the skull by the force of the nail and that there may now be an intracranial injury during removal. The detailed inspection of the head wound shows that the wool cap is indeed deeply embedded in the wound located in the parietal area (sutures and fontanelles are free and do not suggest increased intracranial pressure). The wool cap cannot be removed by careful manipulation. Although a radiographic imaging would be desirable, it is impossible. The nearest computed tomograph is a day's journey away. Since a skull x-ray is not indicated due to the lack of radiodensity of the foreign body, we are not bothered by the fact that no x-ray can be taken in the hospital on this day anyway. The probability that a sharp nail could displace part of the wool into the skull seems very low to me. Nevertheless, we make all the preparations and bring the child into the operating room. With local anesthesia, the wound is slightly enlarged and the wool cap is removed under visual control. There is no bleeding to the outside. A few moments after the removal of the foreign body, the child loses consciousness, shows a bilateral gaze deviation directed cranially and a flaccid tone. Breathing and circulation remain stable; the airways are well open after lateral positioning. We transfer the child to the intensive care unit for further monitoring, where he shows first spontaneous movements upon arrival. The awakening phase is prolonged. When I come to the intensive care unit the next day, the mother is sitting with the awake child in her arms on the bench in front of the intensive care unit and looking into the green of the nearby bush forest. The child also shows no neurological deficits on a detailed clinical examination. After we observe the child for a few more hours, he can be discharged. The wool cap, which only sustained minor damage in this incident, is also taken by the mother. Still not understanding what happened, I watch them leave the hospital and make their way home.

To this day, I do not understand how a sharp object like a nail could have displaced a soft material such as wool through
The skull into the neurocranium. Although we could not prove this to be the case due to the lack of imaging, the acute disturbance of consciousness after removal of the wool cap made this highly likely. The pathophysiological cause of the disturbance of consciousness remained completely unexplained. Perhaps a small bleed occurred after removal of the foreign body, the cortex was irritated, or (non-convulsive) seizures were triggered. A cranial computed tomography scan would have certainly provided some insight here. However, at that time, there were only two computed tomographs in all of Tanzania—one in the capital Dar es Salaam and one in the northern city of Moshi. Both cities were at least a day's journey away—conditions that are quite typical for Africa [1, 2]. Furthermore, the family could not even afford the treatment costs in the hospital, let alone the possible transport of the patient to the computed tomograph and the costs of the examination.

I am glad that in this situation we took the (for me at that time highly unlikely) concerns of the surgeon seriously and removed the foreign body in the operating room and with the best possible view after enlarging the wound. This way we did the best possible under the given circumstances, because there is nothing that does not exist!

25.1 Conclusion

Being a doctor in a low-income country is a special challenge in order to help as many people as possible with few resources. Although one can often compensate for a lack of material and technology with improvisational talent at least to some extent, but if, for example, an oxygen generator fails, then the inspiratory oxygen fraction inhaled by the patient will inevitably fall if there is no oxygen cylinder as a back-up oxygen source. In daily work, the unimaginable poverty of the people on site is evident, but at the same time their unimaginable gratitude and resilience to overcome even terrible fates. In the case described here, it was necessary to weigh the therapeutic options in order to be able to help in the best possible way— fortunately, local wound care was sufficient, as a penetrating head injury would have meant a land transport of about 500 km (311 miles) on bad roads to the nearest neurosurgical treatment with an uncertain outcome.

References

1. Baelani I, Jochberger S, Laimer T, Rex C, Baker T, Wilson IH, Grander W, Dünser MW (2012) Identifying resource needs for sepsis care and guideline implementation in the Democratic Republic of the Congo: a cluster survey of 66 hospitals in four eastern provinces. Middle East J Anaesthesiol 21:559–575
2. Jochberger S, Ismailova F, Lederer W, Mayr VD, Luckner G, Wenzel V, Ulmer H, Hasibeder WR, Dünser MW (2008) „Helfen Berührt" study team. Anesthesia and its allied disciplines in the developing world: a nationwide survey of the Republic of Zambia. Anesth Analg 106:942–948

Resuscitation of an Elderly Patient

Volker Wenzel

▶ What to do when death has already occurred, but then life suddenly shows up again where none should have been anymore? This case shows that there are phenomena in medicine that one cannot sufficiently explain with scientific approaches and research yet.

I was a medical student and earned some money for Medical School as an emergency medical technician in an EMS station. In addition, it was a good opportunity to see (emergency medical) reality up close, which I often missed in the partly very dry examination material with multiple-choice questions in Medical School. The following happened at that time: After hours of waiting for scene calls in the EMS station in the countryside, an alarm comes for our ambulance in a village about 5 km (3 miles) away: "Person collapsed, unresponsive"; a physician-manned ambulance is also alarmed. This mission indication can be anything: people who fell after too much alcohol and really could not get up anymore, homeless people who were asleep, but also patients with a severe stroke. However, the family member who instructed us in front of the emergency site had pure fear in his face—this looked like a very serious situation. We know that the crew of the physician-manned ambulance would arrive at the emergency site about 20 min after us and we would be first of all on our own. We are trained in inserting an intravenous access, intubation and defibrillation but not drug administration, but of course we have hardly any daily routine in these activities—in this respect, a physician is always necessary in a cardiopulmonary resuscitation attempt. The older patient is lying in the bathroom on the first floor under the washbasin. The

V. Wenzel (✉)

Department of Anesthesiology, Intensive Care, Emergency Medicine, and Pain Therapy, Friedrichshafen Regional Medical Center and Tettnang Hospital, Friedrichshafen, Germany
e-mail: v.wenzel@klinikum-fn.de

V. Wenzel (ed.), *Case Studies in Emergency Medicine*,
https://doi.org/10.1007/978-3-662-67249-5_26

situation is clear to us at first sight—sudden circulatory arrest, which requires immediate cardiopulmonary resuscitation. We ask the relatives to leave the bathroom and ask them to call the emergency number 112 again and confirm to the EMS control center that we have initiated cardiopulmonary resuscitation and that the physician-manned ambulance is urgently required; to save time an EMS helicopter was dispatched. Cardiopulmonary resuscitation proceeds smoothly, but we cannot restore spontaneous circulation in the patient. Then something unexpected happens—suddenly the patient's family physician shows up in the bathroom, whom the relatives probably also called in their fear for their grandmother's life. After a short explanation from us (20 min of cardiopulmonary resuscitation with defibrillation without restoring spontaneous circulation), the family physician says: "It makes no sense anymore—please stop cardiopulmonary resuscitation!" We tell the family physician that we should then cancel the EMS helicopter; I am sent by the family phsician to the telephone in the basement. In the living room I tell the relatives that their grandmother did not survive the cardiac arrest despite all efforts. Then I call the emergency number 112 to inform the EMS control center about the family physician's decision to stop cardiopulmonary resuscitation and that the EMS helicopter is no longer needed—the death certificate is to be issued by the family physician. The dispatcher of the rescue control center then orders the EMS helicopter back to the base—but it is already just before landing next to the fruit garden and blows all the flowers off the cherry trees by the downwash of the rotor when it turns around. Then I go back to the bathroom on the first floor to my ambulance colleague and the family physician of our patient. To my surprise, we have to find out that the patient starts breathing again—with a low frequency, but there is no doubt. We can also feel a pulse—the family physician says "It's over soon.", but we are completely overwhelmed—first we determine the death of a patient, but then that's not true?! We discuss with the family physician what we should do, but after a short time and further detailed examination it is clear—the patient breathes regularly and has a stable circulation. We prepare for a transfer to the hospital and the family physician says: "I can't accompany the patient to the hospital, you have to do that yourself!" We reply that we are not allowed to do this as ambulance personnel with such a critically ill patient and suggest that we ask for a physician-manned ambulance from the EMS control center. Again I am sent by the family physician to the living room to make a phone call- at that time, mobile phones did not exist. I tell the relatives that the determination of death was an incredibly embarrassing misunderstanding to me, and that we would now transport the patient to the hospital. The dispatcher of the EMS control center is obviously surprised by the short description of the situation and sends us the previously canceled EMS helicopter again. The EMS helicopter's emergency physician feels quite brusque because of the request, cancellation and re-request, but immediately realizes that a detailed discussion is completely pointless; we then transport the patient to the nearest hospital with him. There the patient is immediately transferred to the intensive care unit, where she dies two weeks later without ever regaining consciousness.

Discussion

In extremely rare cases, it can happen that after the termination of a correctly performed cardiopulmonary resuscitation attempt, spontaneous circulation resumes—but in our analysis over a period of about 15 years in Germany, Austria and Switzerland, not a single cardiopulmonary resuscitated patient survived after such a phenomenon [2]. In a case report of a 55-year-old patient with acute renal failure, cardiopulmonary resuscitation was stopped after 35 min due to persistent asystole. Surprisingly, the patient had a stable circulation again 7 min later and was transported to a hospital where he died three days later from cerebral edema [5]. In this case, it was assumed that renal failure-induced hyperkalemia had caused cardiac arrest and was compensated by sodium bicarbonate infused during cardiopulmonary resuscitation. In another case, a 47-year-old man underwent cardiopulmonary resuscitation. After about 45 min, the resuscitation attempt was stopped due to persistent ventricular fibrillation. 15 min later, a police officer investigating the case discovered that the patient was breathing; he was admitted to the hospital in a stable circulatory condition, but was in a persistent vegetative state and died three months later [3]. The authors could not explain the mechanism in this case, but recommended that after the resuscitation attempt has been completed, the patient should be monitored for about 10–15 min to exclude a Lazarus phenomenon. This case is remarkable because in humans, due to the size of the myocardium, self-defibrillation is actually not possible, as it is in mice or rats. Other possible mechanisms are hypothermia or intoxication. In our analysis [2], we found one case in which the EMS workers mistakenly declared death: A woman (age unknown) tried to commit suicide by taking pills in her Hamburg, Germany apartment. The paramedics called to the scene declared her dead. It was only the undertakers who noticed that the woman was breathing; she survived the incident (Hamburger Morgenpost, 21.02.1997). A 63-year-old woman was pulled lifeless from the Rhine river in Bonn, Germany. After the examination, the emergency physician declared the woman dead. 1½ h later, the undertaker noticed that she was breathing and her heart was beating. However, she died on the same evening (Berliner Kurier, 07.01.2004). Another possible pathomechanism was discussed based on the cardiopulmonary resuscitation attempt of an 81-year-old patient who had to be resuscitated due to a rupture of the A. iliaca externa. Due to the serious underlying disease of a thoracic aortic aneurysm, cardiopulmonary resuscitation was stopped after 25 min and the ventilator was disconnected from the endotracheal tube; about 2 min later, the patient had again stable circulation. He was able to regain normal neurological performance in the following, but died five weeks later [1]. A mechanism was discussed as hyperventilation, which decreases venous return during cardiopulmonary resuscitation by the increased intrathoracic pressure; this would be plausible because after the disconnection of ventilation, circulation was very quickly stabilized again—but the patient also had a pacemaker.

It is unclear why the Lazarus phenomenon of a temporary stable circulation after a terminated cardiopulmonary resuscitation attempt is so rarely described—for this reason, we had an analysis of corresponding reports from the lay press, which brought to light an astonishing number of cases that were unknown in the medical literature. Possible causes could be that the scientific explanations are insufficient, disbelief of the involved EMS workers about the observed phenomenon, often poor and incomplete documentation, fear of missing something and of forensic consequences [4]. Especially because of the case reports from very different health systems in different countries, one must assume that the Lazarus phenomenon exists— it shows that the path between life and death does sometimes not work like a light switch, but sometimes there is another way than one thinks—which can cause a hellish shock for the EMS workers, which of course can quickly call into question the professionalism and expertise of the involved EMS workers and emergency physician.

26.1 Conclusion

Before terminating cardiopulmonary resuscitation attempt, remember that the Lazarus phenomenon exists and exclude possible causes such as hypothermia, intoxication, pulmonary hyperinflation, hypovolemia and bradycardia. After the end of CPR, the patient should be monitored for about 10–15 min; only then should the entry of death be communicated to the relatives.

References

1. Duck MH, Paul M, Wixforth J, Kammerer H (2003) The Lazarus phenomenon. Spontaneous return of circulation after unsuccessful intraoperative resuscitation in a patient with a pacemaker. Anaesthesist 52:413–418
2. Herff H, Loosen SJ, Paal P, Mitterlechner T, Rabl W, Wenzel V (2010) False positive death certification. Does the Lazarus phenomenon partly explain false positive death certification by rescue services in Germany, Austria and Switzerland? Anaesthesist 59:342–346
3. Kamarainen A, Virkkunen I, Holopainen L, Erkkila EP, Yli-Hankala A, Tenhunen J (2007) Spontaneous defibrillation after cessation of resuscitation in out-of-hospital cardiac arrest: a case of Lazarus phenomenon. Resuscitation 75:543–546
4. Maeda H, Fujita MQ, Zhu BL, Yukioka H, Shindo M, Quan L, Ishida K (2002) Death following spontaneous recovery from cardiopulmonary arrest in a hospital mortuary: ‚Lazarus phenomenon‘ in a case of alleged medical negligence. Forensic Sci Int 127:82–87
5. Voelckel W, Kroesen G (1996) Unexpected return of cardiac action after termination of cardiopulmonary resuscitation. Resuscitation 32:27–29

Emergency Cricothyroidotomy 27

Sven Wolf

▶ Since MacGyver there has been the myth of emergency cricothyroidotomy with everyday objects like a ballpoint pen. The present case deals with the question of how far this myth has substance in emergency reality.

On a sunny autumn day, an ambulance and a physician-manned ambulance are sent to a 63-year-old patient with the call sign "respiratory distress" from the EMS dispatch center. According to the EMS dispatch center, the patient was hardly comprehensible on the phone, there are no further past medical history hints. Both EMS vehicles arrive at the same time. The door is opened by the neighbor, as the patient is already unresponsive on the living room floor. In general, we expect many bad things in the EMS; but with the full picture of a myxedema with pronounced cyanosis, all 4 rescuers of the deployed vehicles can hardly hide their horror. The face, mouth and eyes of the patient are balloon-like swollen, the tongue bulges out of the mouth like a child's fist. During the initial monitoring (heart rate 89, blood pressure unmeasurable, oxygen saturation 71%, sinus rhythm on ECG), respiratory and ventilation measures are tried without any recognizable success. Neither a finger nor a Guedel tube can be pushed past the tongue, a spiral tube already sticks at the end of the nasal cavity. The mask can be sealed well in the edematous face, but significant ventilation volumes can not be applied despite the maximum raised lower jaw. On the orders of the emergency physician, the surgical instruments are fetched and opened in the meantime. With an estimated 100 kg body weight, the head contour of the approximately 160 cm tall patient leads almost neckless into the trunk, a classic "no-neck"! The larynx is not palpable percutaneously. About 6 min after arrival at the scene, the emergency physician

S. Wolf (✉)
Department of Emergency Medicine, DIAKOVERE Friederikenstift, Hannover, Germany
e-mail: drsvenwolf@web.de

© The Author(s), under exclusive license to Springer-Verlag GmbH, DE, part of Springer Nature 2023
V. Wenzel (ed.), *Case Studies in Emergency Medicine*,
https://doi.org/10.1007/978-3-662-67249-5_27

makes a transverse skin incision about 8 cm long, 3 fingers caudal to the chin with the scalpel. With both index fingers he prepares or rather "wades" through a wide subcutaneous layer of fat to the trachea and larynx. While holding the "situs" with the thumb and index finger spread, he incises the tight band between the ring and cartilage with the right hand, spreads the small opening with a speculum and inserts a 6.5 tube into the trachea. The patient can now be ventilated sufficiently at a lower level. 500 mg steroid, 1 ampoule antihistamine and 2 mg epinephrine are injected via a peripheral access; a stable circulation and ventilation situation develops. The patient dies in the hospital 2 days later with hypoxic brain damage. The background of the myxedema can not be clarified.

A few days later, the following happens: During car repair work in a garage, there is a massive explosion of gasoline fumes. A 47-year-old patient suffers severe burns (3–4° degree) in the area of the head, neck and front chest wall, as well as an inhalation and smoke gas trauma. The competent EMS services of the respective district are tied up in another scene call, so that the EMS control center, due to the expected extended travel time of ambulance and physician-manned ambulance, alarms a local EMS employee from home as a "first responder". This rescuer finds the patient unconscious (Glasgow Coma Scale 3) lying in front of the garage. Face and front neck/chest region show severe, partly leathery charred burns; the vital parameters indicate profund shock (heart rate 108, blood pressure 90/00, flat, slow breathing movements of <8/min). The EMS employee orders the cooling of the burned areas on the neck and chest with tap water by the fire department, which has meanwhile arrived. At the same time, he places a peripheral venous access (14G). Due to the apparently urgent airway and ventilation problem, he decides to intubate. However, due to the burns, even under considerable force, the mouth or jaw opening is only possible to a maximum of 1.5 cm. The subsequent attempted assisted mask ventilation fails due to gross leaks in the mask on the charred skin areas. As a last resort, he then remembers the story of the "ballpoint pen cricothyrotomy" told again and again by various "specialized trainers". It is not difficult for him to palpate the shield and ring cartilage of the slim patient. However, his quite strong attempts to penetrate the leathery soft tissues and the cricothyreoideum ligament (conicum) with 2 different ballpoint pen models are frustrating; fortunately, however, no injury to large vessels occurs. Meanwhile, the physician-manned ambulance arrives; within 5 min, a safe airway is established using a QuickTrach™ -cricothyrotomy set. The patient can be airlifted to a heavy burn center from the nearby hospital of basic care on the same day. After 2 months and 12 surgical interventions, the patient is transferred to a rehabilitation facility.

And one final event: the 71-year-old resident of a nursing home becomes a patient of the EMS as a result of a frontal fall with her face onto a bedside table. Otherwise awake and oriented, she shows a Glasgow Coma Scale of 3 during the initial examination. There are diffuse bruises, lacerations and unstable facial bones in the area of the nose and the zygomatic arch. The mouth can only be opened to about 1.5 cm with firm contact, according to the information of the carers "this has been like that" since a tumor operation on the jaw 1 year ago. The vital parameters are a blood pressure of 110/70 mmHg, a heart rate of 63 and an oxygen saturation with oxygen mask (6 l/min) of 87% with bradypnoea. Due to the deformed facial skull, assisted mask ventilation is only possible to an unsatisfactory extent. Secretions and blood clots are suctioned off through the narrow mouth opening. The emergency physician decides on a classical open-surgical emergency cricothyrotomy. Since the patient is already deeply unconscious, the procedure is carried out without additional anaesthetic sedation. Although the neck contour is very slender and the larynx is already macroscopically well localized, the scalpel placed together with the skin which is anything but tight slips sideways along the thyroid cartilage several times. Only when the paramedic tightens the skin bilaterally does a reasonable transverse skin incision at the level of the cricothyroid ligament (conicum) succeed. However, the skin incision also cuts through a cranial outgrowth of the thyroid gland with corresponding bleeding. This does not impress the emergency physician at all, he incises the conicum ligament and inserts a 6.5 tube. This allows sufficient ventilation of the patient. The significant oozing of blood from the cricothyrotomy wound has to be compressed manually with a compress up to the hospital. There a local exploration of the wound and ligation of a lobe of the thyroid gland is carried out. Clinically and radiologically, the already suspected complex fractures of the middle face and an subarachnoidal haemorrhage are found after the corresponding diagnostics that has to be surgically intervened.

Discussion

If you ask at symposia or workshops among experienced emergency medical personnel for self-performed emergency cricothyrotomies, the number of raised fingers is very limited [6]. Successful "ballpoint pen operators" of an emergency cricothyrotomy are not known to the author, nor are any serious scientific case studies in this regard. The combination of skin and the tough, fibrous membrane between the ring and thyroid cartilage (conicum/cricothyroideum ligament) renders perforation with a standard ballpoint pen almost impossible. Even with a preparation scissors, these layers are hardly penetrable in vivo and on a cadaver [5].

The exclusive use of ballpoint pens to create an alternative airway is and remains a myth that should not be "set in the head" of physicians and EMS personnel. The valuable time for these frustrated attempts is better invested for non-medical personnel in an emergency situation in an attempt to apply at least small air volumes orally or nasally with the head extended (adults). Accurate numbers for pre-hospital emergency cricothyrotomies in the 1980s and 1990s are not known [6]. In any case, these surgical interventions have decreased significantly in recent years, despite new, great technical aids such as QuickTrach™. "Cannot intubate—cannot ventilate" situations now have a much greater importance in training [6]. There are sufficient aids for the "alternative airway" available (laryngeal mask, Kombitubus™, Larynxtubus™, video laryngoscope etc.) [1], which certainly reduce the maximum success pressure, especially for the less experienced "intubator". Nevertheless, the semi- and full-surgical techniques for emergency cricothyrotomy, despite the relatively high possibility of complications (e.g. tracheal injury, significant bleeding, aspiration), remain an indispensable redundancy for ventilated patients with swollen or destroyed upper airways [2]. In the 3 specific cases mentioned above, although not practiced, the primary puncture of the cricothyreoideum (conicum) ligament and jet ventilation with a 13- or 14-G cannula provides a safe bridge for the minutes until definitive cricothyrotomy [3]. Even if the thyroid gland is palpably small and comes to be positioned caudally of the planned incision, the prevalence of a thin, far-reaching thyroid gland lobe (Lobus pyramidalis glandulae thyroideae) is often transverse through the planned incision area (cricothyroideum ligament). Here, good, tried and tested aids such as the QuickTrach™ set offer a safe alternative to the classic full-surgical access with scalpel and speculum [4]. The danger of significant bleeding from skin vessels and incised thyroid gland tissue is also significantly reduced.

27.1 Conclusion

Emergency cricothyrotomy remains an indispensable redundancy for "can not intubate—can not ventilate" scenarios despite modern "alternative airways". It requires quick, targeted action with knowledge of possible complications. Exercises with emergency cricothyrotomy sets, e.g. on a pig carcass or on a corpse, are very time-consuming, but they provide an ideal practical basis. In any case, it is recommended to regularly deal with both the anatomical normal variants (just palpate each ambulance driver) and the instructions for use of the current emergency cricothyrotomy equipment.

References

1. Buonopane CE, Pasta V, Sottile D, Del Vecchio L, Maturo A, Merola R, Oanunzi A, Urciuoli P, D'Orazi V (2014) Cricothyrotomie performed with the Melker™ set or the QuickTrach® kit: procedure times, learning curves and operators' preference. J Chir 35(7–8):165–170
2. De Koning Gans JM, Zwart DL, Kalkman JC (2010) Acute upper-airway obstructions in primary care. Cricithyrotomie performed by the general practitioner. Ned Tijdschr Geneeskd 154:A1299
3. Hess T, Stuhr M, Knacke PG, Reifferscheid F, Kerner T (2014) Invasive emergency techniques – cricothyroidektomie. Anasthesiol Intensivmed Notfallmed Schmerzther 49(4):230–236
4. Mabry RL, Nichols MC, Shiner DC, Bolleter S, Frankfurt A (2014) A comparison of two open surgical cricothyroidotomy techniques by military medics using a cadaver modell. Ann Emerg Med 63(1):1–5
5. Senthiulkumaran S, David SS, Jena NN, Thirumalaikolundusubramanian P (2014) Cricothyroidotomy and ventilation: physics and physology. J Emerg Med 47(5):131
6. Wong DT, Metha A, Tam AD, Yau B, Wong J (2014) A survey of Canadian anaesthesiologists preferences in difficult intubation and „cannot intubate, cannot ventilate" situations. Can J Anaesth 61(8):717–726

65-Year-old Patient with Shortness of Breath

28

Luise Schnitzer

▶ "Achieve a lot with very little" and "look closely and take seriously" are 2 central themes of this case, which is about taking a holistic view of things.

Home nursing care alarmed us because a COPD patient—permanently dependent on home oxygen—had developed increasing shortness of breath and had become cyanotic. Upon arrival, we find a 65-year-old patient. The room is darkened, the obese gentleman is sitting in bed and greets us friendly and in a good mood. This is striking because people who suffer shortness of breath are usually considerably strained and there is only little room for "politeness" because all focus is concentrated on breathing. The respiratory rate of only 16/min is also striking. We give him a little more oxygen through a nasal cannula, but he remains deeply cyanotic. However, when asked, he reports that he feels as good or as bad as always and cannot report any change in his condition.

My confusion is increasing! Why were we called if his condition is unchanged? Why is he so "cyanotic"? The nurse now reports that she found the patient cyanotic during her daily routine visit and called the fire department despite his protests. A physical examination reveals gurgling and whistling over the lungs as well as coarse rattling noises, the oxygen saturation is 95%, he can cough well, whereupon the coarse rattling noises become less. He has no fever. His skin is blue all over and livid, the fingernails are inconspicuous, but his fingers and hands are blue. Now I am wholly confused. I can only find a somewhat absurd explanation for the cyanosis and point to the bed linen. It is patterned in different shades of blue, it is summer and warm outside, the room is darkened. The patient finds

L. Schnitzer (✉)
Charité University Medicine Berlin, Campus Benjamin Franklin, Department of Cardiology and Pulmology, Berlin, Germany
e-mail: l.schnitzer@gmx.de

© The Author(s), under exclusive license to Springer-Verlag GmbH, DE, part of Springer Nature 2023
V. Wenzel (ed.), *Case Studies in Emergency Medicine*,
https://doi.org/10.1007/978-3-662-67249-5_28

my explanation amusing, my EMS assistant more or less holds his breath and the nurse is extremely skeptical, but cannot and does not want to accept my explanation. Myself a little unsure about my daring diagnosis, I fetch a wet washcloth with soap and can easily remove the "cyanosis". Relieved to have helped the patient and the nurse so quickly and effectively, we leave in a good mood, the patient remains with his speechless nurse in his familiar environment. The first only necessary measure resulting is that the new bed linen is to be washed.

Discussion

Sometimes it's that easy: Although this case is an extremely unusual anecdote, it shows that sometimes a little lateral thinking can be helpful. As an emergency physician, you sometimes come across findings that are not immediately explainable [1]. This is relatively typical in cases of intoxication or drug abuse, especially when patients and relatives deny any abuse. What is decisive are not the statements of third parties or the patient, but the objective condition of the patient, which -in our case- apparently showed a considerable discrepancy to the apparent finding of cyanosis. However, unclear relationships are rarely as easy to clarify as in our patient. Nevertheless, it is always necessary to admit a patient to the hospital, even if only a trivial disease is suspected, be it to reassure yourself or to avoid a long and perhaps fruitless conversation due to lack of time. This is particularly true for patients who have a psychosomatic background and who may not be willing to accept this. The access to the patient is then doubly complicated if in the past there was an actual disease with similar symptoms. This will be demonstrated by another example.

A 32-year-old young woman suffers from an anterior wall infarction due to obstruction of the ramus interventricularis anterior with otherwise uneventful coronary arteries. The damage can be kept small with quick treatment with cardiac catheterization and stent implantation. In the subsequent rehabilitation phase, the patient is doing well and she can cope well with the stress. The difficulties begin when the patient is back at home—without the layer of security that physicians and nursing staff nearby offer, apparently typical angina pectoris complaints occur. She presents herself in the emergency department of the hospital, blood tests and a cardiac catheterization are performed again, which show an uneventful finding. Nevertheless, the patient appears almost weekly with the typical complaints, she is examined, the laboratory values are uneventful and she is discharged home again. Only after the 3rd cardiac catheterization, the treatments are reduced to an ECG and laboratory tests during further visits to the emergency department— ischemia was excluded each time. However, the patient's suffering does not end. Only after 9 months, the patient is recommended a psychotherapeutic treatment, which puts her understandable fears in the foreground. She has two small children and the idea of having a heart that no longer works, possibly dying soon and leaving the children unsupervised, puts the patient to.

After she can also express her concerns, the frequency of angina pectoris attacks drops sharply. Already after 2 weeks she neither calls the number at EMS dispatch doctor, nor does she appear in the hospital herself and has now been symptom-free for more than 4 years. Regular visits to the cardiologist do not reveal any indications of coronary sclerosis, she continues to do sports and is confident in her performance.

28.1 Conclusion

Emergency calls can have very strange causes. Even if the emergency call for help seems completely unfounded, it is important to take the patient's or his relatives' and caregivers' concerns and fears seriously and initiate or help to organize appropriate help. Psychosocial emergencies are a rapidly growing segment of emergency calls, which many emergency physicians find difficult to deal with because they are primarily trained to treat invasively—here, however, one can help a lot with very little.

References

1. Kosan geb. Bathe J (2012) Notarzteinsätze in Alten- und Pflegeheimen – der physician-manned ambulance als Lückenbüßer. Dissertation. Medizinische Fakultät Charité, Universitätsmedizin Berlin

Martin Dünser

▶ The knowledge of the characteristics of a disease is essential for the diagnosis and treatment—but, as this case shows, not always given and self-evident. Even a corresponding treatment option, as shown here, is not self-evident and can have fatal consequences for the patient.

Somewhere in a yurt in the steppe of Mongolia (about four and a half times as large as Germany, but only about 3.2 million inhabitants): A 45-year-old man with a known, poorly controlled epilepsy (antiepileptic medication is only sporadically available) and weekly grand mal seizures has been showing an increase in seizure frequency for a few days. One morning the patient is no longer arousable. A doctor called in from the next village examines the patient and, based on the disturbance of consciousness without recognizable tonic-clonic seizure activity, suspects an intracranial bleed. He recommends, due to the lack of therapeutic consequences (the next hospital with computed tomography or neurosurgery is 700 km (435 miles) away) and the increased risk of transport on unpaved roads, to leave the patient on site in the yurt. The patient's state of consciousness does not change after 2 days, so the family decides to take him by car to the 200 km (124 miles) distant provincial hospital. These distances are hardly imaginable for us, but Mongolia is, after the Western Sahara and Greenland, the world's most sparsely populated country. After more than 12 hours of driving under anything but gentle conditions, the patient reaches the provincial hospital. There he is admitted to the medical ward. A neurological department or a neurologist is not available. The treating physicians also assumed that a spontaneous intracranial bleed

M. Dünser (✉)
Department of Anesthesiology and Critical Care Medicine, Kepler University Hospital, Linz, Austria
e-mail: Martin.Duenser@kepleruniklinikum.at

© The Author(s), under exclusive license to Springer-Verlag GmbH, DE, part of Springer Nature 2023
V. Wenzel (ed.), *Case Studies in Emergency Medicine*,
https://doi.org/10.1007/978-3-662-67249-5_29

(e.g. an intracerebral hypertensive mass bleed) was most likely to explain the patient's coma. The therapy is purely supportive—lateral position, oxygen administration, and so on. Further intensive care is impossible due to the lack of equipment, the lack of experienced personnel and the lack of space for an intensive care unit. At the insistence of the relatives, the physicians agree to transfer the patient who continues to be in coma to the university hospital in the Mongolian capital Ulaanbaatar. The transport—this time 200 km (124 miles) of the total 500 km (311 miles) on paved roads—is again carried out by private car. On the 6th day after the onset of consciousness, the patient arrives in the emergency room of the university hospital. A short time later I am involved to evaluate the admission to the intensive care unit. Clinically, the patient shows a Glasgow Coma Scale of 5 (eyes 1, verbal 1, motor 3). The muscle reflexes are barely perceptible at all extremities, the Babinski reflex is weakly elicitable bilaterally. The pupils are medium-wide and react only slowly to light. On passive opening of the eyelids, a weak, rhythmic twitching can be seen at the lower eyelid. Based on the history of the family and clinical presentation, the diagnosis of a non-convulsive status epilepticus is very likely. Differential diagnoses include a brain (stem) hemorrhage or -ischemia as well as a metabolic coma cause. After a cranial computed tomogram (the university hospital is one of the few hospitals in Mongolia at this time that has a computed tomograph), which shows signs of brain edema, an EEG is performed. This shows the picture of a status epilepticus with a clear slowing of the background rhythm up to phases of a burst suppression. Together with the neurologist, we administer a total of 30 mg diazepam as well as carbamazepine and phenytoin. A further escalation of the antiepileptic therapy, as provided for in the stepwise algorithm for the treatment of status epilepticus, is not possible. In addition to carbamazepine and phenytoin, no other antiepileptic substances are available. Since the patient's prognosis is judged to be very unfavorable due to the long delay until antiepileptic therapy was started and the evolving brain edema, we decide that another patient (32 years, septic shock with peritonitis due to a perforated appendicitis) is admitted to the intensive care unit bed with the possibility for mechanical ventilation. This renders induction of a barbiturate coma, which requires endotracheal intubation, impossible. The patient is treated on an intensive care bed without the possibility for mechanical ventilation for another 5 days. His state of consciousness does not change, but deteriorates step by step. In the end, the patient has a Glasgow Coma Scale of 3. Since the chances of neurological recovery are considered to be extremely low by all team members and several other patients are waiting for intensive care unit admission, the patient is transferred to the neurological ward for further care. I visit him there a few days later. His condition remains unchanged. He dies shortly thereafter.

Discussion
Non-convulsive status epilepticus is a common, although often unrecognized, cause of altered consciousness. For all those, like the initial physicians involved in this case, who have hitherto associated epilepsy necessarily

with tonic-clonic focal or generalized seizure forms, this diagnosis does not exist. Thus, the correct therapy is not administered, which—as in our case example—can end fatally. Non-convulsive seizure forms were first described by Lennox in 1945 [1] and considered a rare event for many years. First prevalence studies in the 1970s suggested that non-convulsive status epileptici made up approximately 25% of all status forms [2]. Today we know that non-convulsive seizures are very common in older people with vigilance disorders (up to 30%). It is important to know that approximately 25% of convulsive states transition into a non-convulsive status epilepticus after the cessation of the tonic-clonic movement component (e.g. due to medication). In addition to subtle clinical seizure clues (e.g. rhythmic twitching of the eyelids during passive opening), persistent coma despite tonic-clonic seizure symptoms have abated should be considered as a potential indicator of non-convulsive status epilepticus [3]. If there is reasonable suspicion, this can only be confirmed or ruled out by EEG. The most common causes of non-convulsive status epilepticus are similar to those of convulsive status epilepticus and include ischemia/trauma, inadequate treatment of known epilepsy, medications/withdrawal, metabolic influences (sepsis to intoxication), neurodegenerative processes, central nervous system infections, and neoplasms. Identifying the cause of status epilepticus is essential and a prerequisite for successful therapy. Antiepileptic treatment of non-convulsive status epilepticus does not differ from that of convulsive status epilepticus. However, the two seizure forms differ in their response to antiepileptic therapy. While refractory convulsive states (no response to first-line, i.e. benzodiazepines, and second-line, i.e. phenytoin, levetiracetam or valproate, therapies) are observed in approximately ¼ of cases, refractory seizure patterns have been described in up to 90% of non-convulsive states [4].

In our case, it was most likely a deterioration of idiopathic epilepsy due to inadequate antiepileptic therapy. The presented case impressively shows how crucial knowledge of the existence of a non-convulsive seizure can be and what consequences the failure to recognize this form of epilepsy can have. In 2004—when I was involved in the treatment of this patient—the knowledge of non-convulsive status epilepticus in Mongolian medical circles was only rudimentary. One of the main reasons for this is probably the lack of availability of EEG machines in most hospitals. The university hospital was one of three hospitals in the Mongolian capital Ulaanbaatar (approx. 1.3 million inhabitants) that had such a device at that time.

29.1 Conclusion

The suspected diagnosis of spontaneous intracerebral hemorrhage (e.g. hypertensive mass bleeding) made by the treating physicians was unlikely in view of the past medical history and presented clinical picture, even though intracerebral hemorrhage was one of the most frequent causes of sudden non-traumatic loss of consciousness in persons >40 years in Mongolia. A high prevalence of untreated arterial hypertension among the Mongolian population is likely to explain this. The fact that the loss of consciousness due to the non-convulsive seizure occurred in this patient outside the Mongolian capital, immensely worsened the chances of treatment and healing of the patient. In 2004, intensive care was hardly existent in Mongolia outside of Ulaanbaatar. Poor transport links and long distances without existing transport facilities (e.g. ground or air-based transfer options for critically ill patients) represented additional adverse factors. Within the last 15 years, Mongolia has experienced a significant improvement in its road and transport network as well as the availability of EEG devices as part of its economic upturn.

References

1. Lennox WG (1945) The petit mal epilepsies: their treatment with tridione. JAMA 129:1069–1074
2. Celesia GG (1976) Modern concepts of status epilepticus. JAMA 325:1571–1574
3. Al-Mufti F, Claassen J (2014) Neurocritical care: status epilepticus review. Crit Care Clin 30:751–764
4. Mayer SA, Claassen J, Lokin J et al (2002) Refractory status epilepticus: frequency, risk factors, and impact on outcome. Arch Neurol 59:205–210

A Pale Patient

30

Frank Marx

▶ How to react when 2 lives are at stake and it is not initially clear what the situation can be attributed to? And how to deal with the relatives when a world collapses from one moment to the next? This case impressively shows how important the topic of psychohygiene can be for the emergency doctor.

On a November afternoon, the crew of an ambulance is ordered to transport a pregnant patient in labor to the hospital as part of a planned admission. When the employees see the patient in her apartment, she is strikingly pale and reports severe back pain that is continuously present and getting worse. The husband of the patient, who is a physician himself, and the couple's 6-year-old son are still present in the apartment on the second floor of a multi-family house. When trying to transfer the patient from the living room sofa to the prepared stretcher, she collapses lifeless. While the paramedic immediately begins cardiopulmonary resuscitation, the rescue worker runs back to his ambulance to request an emergency doctor.

At the time of the EMS dispatch, I am as the medical director of the ambulance service by chance only about 3 streets away from the scene of the accident. I decide to drive to the scene of the accident in addition to the requested emergency physician and see upon entering the apartment, a woman about 30 years old lying on the floor in the living room. Cardiac compressions and ventilation are continuously performed since the collapse of circulation. The husband states that his wife is in the 39th week of pregnancy; during the initial examination, I notice that the woman is very pale. The pupils are maximally dilated and not round. While I try

F. Marx (✉)
Intensive Care Helicopter Christoph Giessen, Malteser Hilfsdienst Diözese Münster,
Giessen / Münster, Germany
e-mail: drmarx@web.de

to create a venous access on the forearm, I ask the husband to call the EMS control center again at the emergency number 112. The dispatcher receives a precise location report from me and I ask him to send a gynecologist and a surgeon for an emergency Cesarean section from a nearby hospital to the scene of the accident. I can not puncture a peripheral vein and so I perform a venous puncture of the V. jugularis interna with an 18G cannula. This succeeds without problems and I inject infusion solutions and adrenaline through this access. I make sure that the pregnant woman's abdomen is turned to the left to avoid a reduction of venous return during cardiopulmonary resuscitation [4]. Meanwhile, an ambulance has arrived and the paramedics retrieve additional emergency medical equipment from the vehicle, including surgical instruments. Everything is prepared for the emergency Cesarean section during cardiopulmonary resuscitation. About 10 min after the alarm, a gynecological assistant with advanced training and a specialist in surgery arrive in the apartment. I briefly explain the situation and ask the gynecological colleague to perform an emergency Cesarean section. However, he hesitates and is not convinced by me to do this immediately. Instead, he calls his chief physician from the nearby hospital and he advises him not to perform the procedure on site. The already intubated patient is therefore brought to the ambulance during ongoing cardiopulmonary resuscitation and transported to the hospital 4 min away. There, an ultrasound is performed and it is determined that there are no fetal heart tones; at this time the resuscitation attempt has been going on already for 40 min. As a result, resuscitation efforts are discontinued.

The patient's husband is waiting in the waiting area outside the emergency room. I report to him the sad news of the death of his wife and his child. He leans on me, cries and sobs: "You're a physician as well, can you understand what I'm feeling right now?" During the whole operation I was the organizer, the decision maker and I made decisions and followed them up in a targeted manner—but here, certainly also by the physical proximity to this weeping, completely desperate man, I struggle with tears. At the autopsy of the corpse it turns out that there has been a rupture of the abdominal aorta; accordingly, there are considerable amounts of blood in the abdomen.

Discussion

In this case, all the promising conditions that can be present in a cardiopulmonary resuscitation came together at first: trained staff of the ambulance service immediately started cardiopulmonary resuscitation of the patient [6] when she suffered a circulatory collapse and the first physician was on site within 2 min of the event. An emergency medical vehicle supported with additional personnel and with the material required for an emergency Cesarean section arrived within 10 min, bringing along a gynecologist and a surgeon. The hospital with the department of gynecology and obstetrics was only 4 min drive from the scene of the accident. There were several vehicles of the ambulance service and the fire department at the scene of the accident; the transport of the patient up the stairs to the ambulance took no longer than 2 min even during resuscitation efforts. Although this sequence represents an amazing speed of the rescue measures, it was still not fast enough. An analysis of maternal circulatory arrest during pregnancy showed that the emergency Cesarean section should have been performed within 4 min of the event in order to achieve the optimum survival probability for the child [3], which is practically only possible in the hospital. Even if these numbers from the 1980s are cautiously considered due to the medical progress, they are confirmed by current data. In a Swedish case series, neither mother nor child could be saved by an emergency Cesarean section after 30 min of CPR; in contrast, after 6 min of cardiopulmonary resuscitation, both the child and the mother could be saved by an emergency Cesarean section. In another patient in the 39th week of pregnancy with spontaneous aortic rupture, an emergency Cesarean section was performed after 10 min of cardiopulmonary resuscitation; the child survived, but the mother died [8]. These experiences show that our patient and her unborn child had no chance of survival when realistically considered.

The patient's conspicuous pallor already made me suspicious at the first examination. The patient's husband watched our resuscitation efforts, venipuncture, intubation, repetitive injections of epinephrine and ongoing cardiopulmonary resuscitation from the hallway with the son—as a medical colleague, he certainly immediately correctly assessed that the situation was almost hopeless. At no time during the cardiopulmonary resuscitation over 40 min did ventricular fibrillation occur; the patient remained in asystole until the end of the resuscitation attempt—a sign that the patient was probably completely bled out. With the arrival of the gynecological and surgical colleagues, I would have expected an immediate laparotomy or emergency section and was initially frustrated by his refusal to perform the laparotomy and develop the child. Retrospectively, with the collapse of the patient's circulation, her death and the death of her child were determined by the uncontrollable, intra-abdominal bleeding caused by a completely ruptured aortic aneurysm. No matter how efficient cardiopulmonary resuscitation was and no matter how excellent the team worked, they could not have saved the child and the mother—even if the aneurysm had ruptured in the hospital, it would not have been certain that these 2 lives could have been saved. About 50% of aortic ruptures in women under 40 years of age occur during pregnancy. It was unknown whether our patient suffered from a vascular disorder such as Marfan syndrome, which predisposes to an aortic rupture [1]; but even in pregnant women without cardiovascular pathology, fatal ruptures of the aorta have been described [7]. In a Dutch study, only 13 maternal deaths due to aortic rupture were described in over 3 million births, which shows the extremely low risk (approx. 1:240,000) [5]—but even that was only a weak consolation for the husband and son of this patient.

The technical and organizational aspects of cardiopulmonary resuscitation are a trained procedure; dealing with relatives is more difficult for the treating emergency physician, but certainly also for the other rescue workers involved. While many professions use Balint groups [2] and similar discussion groups for reflection, this is very rare in the emergency medical field. It would be helpful to carry out supervision for emergency physicians in order to enable the emergency physician, but also the other involved forces, to carry out psychohygiene on the one hand, but also to enable them to appropriately respond to the patient, relatives and colleagues in extreme situations. It should also be mentioned that the professional processing in the context of a case discussion also helps to reflect and optimize one's own decisions.

30.1 Conclusion

Aortic ruptures in pregnant women without vascular pathology are extremely rare, but end with a very high probability of death if the rupture is complete—even if resuscitation measures are taken very quickly. An emergency Cesarean section can theoretically also save the child during ongoing cardiopulmonary resuscitation, but must be carried out within a few minutes, which is almost impossible in the EMS. Emergency physicians should be aware that they will experience medically dramatic and emotionally extremely stressful missions and should therefore not hesitate to work out stressful situations in Balint groups.

References

1. Birsner ML, Farber JL, Berghella V (2008) Fatal aortic dissection in a patient with a family history of Marfan syndrome. Obstet Gynecol 112:472–475
2. Hafner S, Otten H, Petzold ER (2011) Balint group work in Germany – results from a survey of Balint group leaders. Z Psychosom Med Psychother 57:233–243
3. Katz VL, Dotters DJ, Droegemueller W (1986) Perimortem cesarean delivery. Obstet Gynecol 68:571–576
4. Kinsella SM (2003) Lateral tilt for pregnant women: why 15 degrees? Anaesthesia 58:835–836
5. la Chapelle CF, Schutte JM, Schuitemaker NW, Steegers EA, van Roosmalen J (2012) Maternal mortality attributable to vascular dissection and rupture in the Netherlands: a nationwide confidential enquiry. BJOG 119:86–93
6. Nolan JP, Soar J, Wenzel V, Paal P (2012) Cardiopulmonary resuscitation and management of cardiac arrest. Nat Rev Cardiol 9:499–511
7. Srettabunjong S (2013) Spontaneous rupture of acute ascending aortic dissection in a young pregnant woman: a sudden unexpected death. Forensic Sci Int 232:e5–8
8. Zdolsek HJ, Holmgren S, Wedenberg K, Lennmarken C (2009) Circulatory arrest in late pregnancy: caesarean section a vital decision for both mother and child. Acta Anaesthesiol Scand 53:828–829

Collapse During Seniors' Hike

31

Joachim Koppenberg

▶ This case shows that not only the place of use requires full concentration from the EMS team, but also the handover to the emergency team in the hospital: The patient remains in the responsibility of the deployment team until a clear "Your patient!" has been said.

The follow-up deployment reaches us on the return flight from the hospital to our Swiss Alpine base in the Engadin. I am just enjoying the fantastic panorama of the mountains at sunset after a sunny and eventful summer day—despite the now over 15 years of experience in air rescue. Via radio we receive the message that it is a "collapse" of a hiker in the border area between Austria and Switzerland—flight time approximately 9 min. The deployment site is located at approximately 1.400 m / 4,600 feet above sea level on an idyllic high plateau with a small mountain lake, so that we can land near the deployment site without any problems. There is an English hiking group of six seniors accompanied by a local hiking guide who can give detailed information. The patient is a 67-year-old British woman who was able to keep up with the previous hike of approximately 6 h without any problems and did not stand out in particular. For about 30 min she has now been complaining of discomfort and exhaustion, but at first this was associated with the declining condition. Only when she could really no longer walk and lost consciousness for a short time on each occasion was an emergency call made. The hiking guide brought her into the stable side position— breathing was always present. The patient is now lying on a rescue blanket and does not look fit at all— pale and sweaty. She is awake and responds to closed questions with yes or no,

J. Koppenberg (✉)
Department of Anesthesiology, Pain Therapy and Emergency Medicine,
Center da sanda Engiadina Bassa, Scuol, Switzerland
e-mail: Joachim.Koppenberg@cseb.ch

V. Wenzel (ed.), *Case Studies in Emergency Medicine*,
https://doi.org/10.1007/978-3-662-67249-5_31

but according to the hiking guide, the level of consciousness changes within a few minutes from completely awake with a GCS of 15 to just awake. I can hardly feel the slow pulse, so I quickly insert a venous access, while the paramedic monitors the patient in parallel. The blood pressure is 78/35 mmHg, the irregular heart rate is slow at 34/min and spontaneous oxygen saturation is 84%. The blood sugar determination shows a normoglycaemia. The analysis of the ECG shows an intermittently occurring AV block III, which can also explain the changing levels of consciousness of the patient. In addition to a rapid oxygen supply with 6 l/min, I explain to the present husband what the current problem of his wife is and that we would have to provide her with an external, transcutaneous pacemaker undergoing analgosedation next. The husband reported that his wife has been treated for years for arterial Hypertension taking a β-blocker, but is otherwise healthy and also well-tolerated. Meanwhile, we have glued the multifunction electrodes for the pacer next to the ECG and drawn up Midazolam and Morphine for sedation and injected the first dose. I set the pacemaker frequency in the VVI mode (demand or demand mode) to 70/min and slowly turn up the power. Already at 45 mA the pacemaker takes over completely (capture), so that I can fix the power at 50 mA with a certain safety margin. Within a few seconds the patient is completely awake, so that I can also explain the working hypothesis and the measures taken personally. The blood pressure now stabilizes at 115/80 mmHg and the oxygen saturation is now 97%. Even if the patient describes the pacemaker impulses as not quite as bad (verbal rating scale = 3–4/10), I deepen analgosedation because the patient does not have to "endure" anything. Once the situation has stabilized, we discuss the transport to the next suitable hospital. It turns out that the hiking group started from Austria and also wants to return there. Since the next hospital is on the Austrian side in the place where the "car-free" couple is also on vacation, it is quickly clear that we will transport the patient to this hospital after pre-registration. After a short information of the Swiss and the Austrian rescue control centers, we load the absolutely stable patient undergoing pacemaker therapy and analgosedation into the helicopter and set off on the approximately 15-minute flight. Such cross-border operations are not unusual in our region, but my joy on this day increases again and it seems to be the perfect conclusion to a perfect day. For a better understanding, I have to add at this point that this is the base hospital of the Austrian emergency helicopter, where I was allowed to work for some years. But since I have not been there for a long time, I secretly hope to meet one or the other "old" colleague from this time in the emergency room. And I should not be disappointed! After an absolutely stable flight we land and with the typical pick-up team at the landing site there is a big "hello". "Nice to see you again— but what kind of weird uniform are you wearing?" Or "Yes, yes, really nice, but you get out of the wrong helicopter!" I immediately feel "at home" again and can therefore also purposefully take the way to the emergency room and the internal admission there. In the emergency room it gets even better: I practically know everyone and almost everyone recognizes me again—a "home game"! And then, of all people, the former colleague whom I got to know and appreciate particularly during the Austrian air rescue comes to hand over. After a first warm welcome,

I concentrate on the most important information about the absolutely stable patient, the mission and finally do not forget to hand over the mobile phone number of the husband who is still on the way back.

We have just started to reminisce about old times and exchange ideas about what the children are up to when the attending nurse suddenly screams and we have to realize that the patient is deeply unconscious. The heart rate on the emergency room monitor shows an irregular heart rate of 34/min, the blood pressure is 65/25 mmHg and the oxygen saturation with 6 l/min is 90%. There are no pacemaker spikes to be found. I immediately turn up the pacemaker's power to maximum strength—but nothing changes. How can that be? First we inject fractionated adrenaline i.v. 0.1 mg-wise until the patient becomes more awake and the heart rate and blood pressure rise slightly. At the same time we feverishly think about what to do. A new external pacemaker is needed, which is quickly brought in from the nearby emergency room. When this is connected and the corresponding current value of 45 mA is reached, an immediate takeover occurs and every pacemaker spike is followed by a QRS complex again. The patient stabilizes promptly and is responsive again. After a short examination by the admitting colleague, the patient is quickly transferred to the intensive care unit for placement of a transvenous pacemaker. The further course is uneventful and the patient can have an internal pacemaker implanted the next day without any problems.

Discussion
After the patients have arrived safely in the intensive care unit, we go through the possible sources of error for the interruption of pacemaker therapy in the emergency room with all participants. The inspection of the devices does not reveal any technical problems. After we have gone through the situation again with the involved emergency room nurse, it suddenly becomes clear to us. While we thought we were done with the transfer, the emergency room nurse started to hang up the monitoring on the emergency room devices as usual and started with the ECG. This resulted in the pacemaker in our device's demand mode receiving feedback ("afferent limb") about the device's own ECG missing, as it was now being derived from the emergency room monitor. Therefore, he simply turned off his "efferent" pacemaker function [1]. When we re-enacted the situation, we also noticed that our device also showed "check ECG electrodes" in the top line—but this went unnoticed in the stressful situation.

In fact, all manufacturers of monitors/defibrillators equipped with an external pacemaker recommend that an ECG is also necessary for the pacemaker function. In principle, pacing could also be carried out exclusively via the multifunction electrodes on some devices, but then an ECG derivation without any detection of the patient's own frequency with a rigid pacemaker frequency in the VOO or non-demand or fixed frequency mode. This is hardly used today and should only be used in extreme emergencies, e.g. when there is no ECG. So if we hadn't had another pacemaker available, we could have switched to the rigid VOO or non-demand or fixed frequency mode until our problem was clarified. Some devices even switch to this emergency mode automatically if the ECG fails, but then have to be switched on again. But this would only be the purely technical solution to a problem that was actually quite different and basically avoidable [2].

The actual "turning point" was somewhere else entirely—namely, the early extinguished attention to the patient due to other, in this case personally motivated priorities after the supposedly completed transfer [3]. This was completed orally, but by no means carried out. In fact, this is a phenomenon that can regularly be observed not only after reaching the emergency room, but also during transfers to the intensive care unit: you have finally reached the supposedly safe environment with sufficient and competent support. Then, in addition to the oral transfer, the monitoring or the infusion pump is hung up in parallel by several people and the patient experiences a longer monitoring break and possibly also a therapy interruption, e.g. of sedatives or even worse of catecholamines. If monitoring is started again, the patient has deteriorated due to the unnoticed and unmonitored therapy interruption (e.g. too awake due to lack of sedation or hypotonic due to insufficient catecholamine infusion) [4]. The taking over colleagues roll their eyes and take over the therapy stressed, while the EMS colleague loudly assures "But the patient was stable until just now!", Which is probably true, but now no one is interested or helpful anymore.

31.1 Conclusion

On the one hand, this case showed me once again that one must first get to know the devices with which one works, including their quirks or "pitfalls", and that one must become familiar not only with their function, but also with the error messages and possibilities (this also includes considering possible "trouble-shoot" scenarios). On the other hand, it was once again made clear to me that the patient is not automatically safe when he or she reaches the emergency room, but that, on the contrary, the handover must be considered a high-risk situation for the patient. Therefore, in addition to a structured oral handover, what is needed above all is attentive and critical accompaniment of the actual patient transfer (repositioning, monitoring, infusion pump therapy, ventilation, etc.). Only when this is completed may the patient be considered "handed over" safely and the responsibility for the patient may be handed over to the emergency room team. Ideally, this is communicated loudly and clearly to all involved: "The handover is complete." or "Your patient!"

References

1. Koppenberg J, von Hintzenstern U (2020) Risikomanagement im Notarztdienst. In: Notarztleitfaden, 9th edn. Urban und Fischer Verlag, München
2. Scholz J, Sefrin P, Böttiger BW et al (2013) Notfallmedizin, 3rd edn. Georg Thieme Verlag, Stuttgart
3. Lendemans S (2012) Interfaces in emergency medicine. Exemplified by treatment of the severely injured. Notf Rettungsmed 15:300–304
4. Siebert R (2009) Strukturierte Patientenübergabe. Star. Life 2:17–21

Serious Kick Injury

Frank Marx

▶ Providing emergency care to patients who are very young often poses a special challenge for rescue workers. And, as this case shows, it is once again necessary to weigh very carefully which subsequent steps might be the right ones.

On a warm autumn day, shortly before we sign off at dusk, we receive a call from a hospital in basic and regular care, located about 15 min flight time away, while we are on duty at the EMS helicopter "Christoph 9" in the city of Duisburg. A 10-year-old child has fallen off a horse and then the horse hit the child's chest with a hoof; the child is unstable and has difficulty breathing. 2 min after the alarm, our EMS helicopter takes off to transport the child to a university hospital. We reach the destination area a short time later and are then driven to the hospital, which is only a few hundred metres away, in an ambulance with our equipment. In the emergency department, surgeons, anaesthetists and nursing staff are caring for the apparently seriously injured child. The chest X-ray shows a haemopneumothorax, which has been relieved by chest drains on the left and right; in addition, there is a suspicion of an aneurysmatic injury to blood vessels near the heart. Only small amounts of blood are draining into the drainage bags via both chest drains. Intravenous anaesthesia is being maintained via peripheral venous accesses. In the language of traumatology, the child therefore has a B and a C problem, because mechanical ventilation requires peak pressures of 50 cm H_2O in order to enable ventilation, and circulation is unstable—only with norepinephrine can a blood pressure of 90 mmHg systolic be achieved. The child has a cyanotic skin colour and the pulse oximetric oxygen saturation is barely 80% with ventilation using

F. Marx (✉)
Intensive Care Helicopter Christoph Giessen, Malteser Hilfsdienst Diözese Münster,
Giessen/Münster, Germany
e-mail: drmarx@web.de

V. Wenzel (ed.), *Case Studies in Emergency Medicine*,
https://doi.org/10.1007/978-3-662-67249-5_32

100% oxygen. The check of the tube position and the chest drains shows a correct position and yet the pulmonary situation is dramatically bad, despite suction of the airways. A transoesophageal echo or computed tomogram is not available. Objectively, the child is not transportable, but the therapy options in the small hospital have been exhausted and correctly carried out. Therefore, I decide to prepare the child for transport to the helicopter.

The child is transferred to our helicopter stretcher and I ventilate it with a breathing bag to which a demand valve is connected, so that I ventilate with pure oxygen. Before take-off, I call the emergency coordinator at the university hospital and notify the child again, which was already registered by the surgical department of the smaller hospital. In the dusk we then take off for the university hospital, which is about 22 min flying time away. I have initially connected the patient to the ventilator in the helicopter. However, high peak pressures and a pulse oximetric oxygen saturation of <70% show to me that I cannot ventilate the child in this way. I paralyze the child again, deepen intravenous anesthesia and change the ventilation parameters several times on the ventilator. However, no change in settings leads to the desired success and I long for the end of the flight because I feel that the situation is deteriorating from minute to minute. There is indeed an arterial pressure measurement, but I cannot achieve a satisfactory signal, which is probably due to vibrations in the helicopter. With the non-invasive blood pressure measurement, I cannot achieve any measurements, the device is constantly measuring, but no results are displayed. I cannot feel a peripheral pulse and I guess a pulse on the A. carotis more than I really feel it. The ECG shows a tachycardic sinus rhythm and the pulse oximetry indicates with a value of about 70% and minimal pulse waves on the monitor that the child actually still has circulation. In capnography, I measure values above 60 mmHg, which supports this assumption. I now set the norepinephrine in the perfusion pump even higher, without really being able to measure an exact systolic blood pressure. Finally, I disconnect the child from the ventilator and ventilate it manually as on the transport to the helicopter. This is difficult for me because I have the impression that I can hardly transport air into the lungs. The ventilation pressures are maximally high and I am far from being able to offer the child a "laminar" air flow. And yet my manual ventilation seems to work better than ventilation with the ventilator, because the pulse oximetric oxygen saturation rises again to values around 80%. So we fly into the dusk and, as planned, reach the university hospital after what seems like an endless 22 min. Usually it takes 2 or 3 min from landing to unloading the patient, because the engines of the EMS helicopter are supposed to cool down in idle mode in order to reduce engine wear. In this case, however, I ask the pilot to shut down the engines immediately. The rotor blades have not yet come to a standstill when the paramedic already gets out and prepares to unload the child. The transport of the stretcher by elevator to the emergency room of the university hospital takes me agonizingly long. The child is still cyanotic, the skin marbled and there is no talk of reasonable cardiorespiratory values. Only capnometry shows high end-tidal carbon dioxide values, which makes me somewhat confident. Pulse oximetrically,

I no longer get any signals in the elevator; I have the feeling that the 10-year-old girl is now dying.

Although I am experienced in the care of emergency patients, I am nevertheless glad that I can hand over the child in the emergency room; after a short examination, the child is taken to the operating room and a thoracotomy is performed. Intraoperatively, there is an injury of several bronchial branches and a large pericardial effusion is relieved. Several ribs are fractured near the sternum. However, an aneurysmatic injury of large vessels, as we suspected from the chest X-ray, is not present. Postoperatively, the child recovers quickly in the next few days. 20 days after the accident, it is transferred to the home hospital and 10 days later discharged home; a longer rehabilitation phase follows and eventually the child makes a full recovery.

Discussion

Injuries of children under 15 years of age while handling horses are probably underestimated, but caused 13,000 admissions per year in US emergency departments in one study. The Injury Severity Score was higher compared to other injury mechanisms, but only in pedestrians hit by cars [1]. Horses can weigh several hundred kg, run up to 50 km/h (31 mph) and suddenly change their running direction or react startledly to noise—all factors that favor a fall. However, regardless of a fall from a horse, additional hip injuries can be very serious, causing severe facial or head injuries [2], cardiac rupture [3] and, as in our case, severe thoracic trauma [4].

Only cardiorespiratory stable patients should be transported with an EMS helicopter to avoid elaborate or impossible measures during transport in the aircraft. Accordingly, one should treat cardiorespiratory unstable patients thoroughly before air transport to spare the helicopter crew coping with precarious situations with difficult conditions during the flight. However, when we stood in the emergency department of the small hospital and this severely injured child was lying in front of us, I came to the conviction that there was no further treatment option on site. The child was, according to Powell et al. [5], in a situation in which a delayed transport to a trauma center and thus a delayed causal therapy makes survival less likely. Especially a transport with an EMS helicopter can help in such a situation to gain life-saving time in a severe thoracic trauma, for example, to enable only at a trauma center possible treatment options such as extracorporeal membrane oxygenation [6].

The chest injuries suggested that serious intrathoracic injuries had led to a tension pneumothorax, but since the two thoracic drains were properly placed and radiologically controlled, I did not know of any other approach to improve the pulmonary situation. The circulatory situation deteriorated increasingly after my arrival at the referring hospital and it might actually have been an option to perform a pericardial puncture—but due to the lack of imaging possibilities this diagnosis could not be made. However, the problem with such punctures is that it is usually not possible to achieve sufficient relief by blood clotting in the pericardium in most cases. Paramedics of the London Air Ambulance have been able to save 11 patients with subsequent good neurological outcome in a total of 71 cases of pre-hospital circulatory collapse after trauma by thoracotomy directly at the accident site; in each of these cases a pericardial tamponade was evacuated. [7]. But our little patient had no circulatory arrest and I would not have dared to take such drastic measures without prior training—even for surgeons this measure is a rare challenge and a high decision hurdle.

What makes such an intervention an event that one will never forget? In this case it was a very moving letter that I received months later from the patient and her mother, accompanied by an invitation to visit her. And when I did that later, I met a completely healthy, now 11-year-old girl who was physically and mentally fully capable and had no memory whatsoever of the accident, the dramatic hours and the strenuous days afterwards. How nice if you can say that as a patient.

32.1 Conclusion

Horse riding accidents can be extremely dangerous. A thoracic trauma can take a dramatic course due to the simultaneous influence on the lung and cardiac function. The decision between stabilization on site and rapid transfer to a trauma center must be weighed carefully in each individual case.

References

1. Jagodzinski T, DeMuri GP (2005) Horse-related injuries in children: a review. WMJ 104:50–54
2. Exadaktylos AK, Eggli S, Inden P, Zimmermann H (2002) Hoof kick injuries in unmounted equestrians. Improving accident analysis and prevention by introducing an accident and emergency based relational database. Emerg Med J 19:573–575
3. Alami A, Slaoui A, Drissi-Kacemi A, Maazouzi W (2003) Right atrial rupture following a hoof kick to the chest wall. J Cardiovasc Surg (Torino) 44:65–66
4. Bruck E, Stiletto R, Botel T, Gotzen L, Moosdorf R, Leppek R (1996) Blunt thoracic trauma with aortic rupture and lung contusion caused by hoof kick in a 15-year-old girl. Diagnostic and therapeutic management. Unfallchirurg 99:901–904
5. Powell DG, Hutton K, King JK, Mark L, McLellan HM, McNab J, Mears D (1997) The impact of a helicopter emergency medical services program on potential morbidity and mortality. Air Med J 16:48–50
6. Voelckel W, Wenzel V, Rieger M, Antretter H, Padosch S, Schobersberger W (1998) Temporary extracorporeal membrane oxygenation in the treatment of acute traumatic lung injury. Can J Anaesth 45:1097–1102
7. Davies GE, Lockey DJ (2011) Thirteen survivors of prehospital thoracotomy for penetrating trauma: a prehospital physician-performed resuscitation procedure that can yield good results. J Trauma 70:E75–E78

Student with Heart Problems

Joachim Koppenberg

▶ "Face your fears" is the motto of this case, which makes it very clear how important it is to face up to a situation or to prepare for it preventively if one is particularly afraid of it, but that too much theoretical knowledge implemented can sometimes also be detrimental to the patient and the treatment.

Each of us probably has our own medical preferences and hobbies, but also our absolute horror scenarios of a call-out. In addition to the child emergencies, which are certainly also the case with many other colleagues, these were long-term patients with cardiac rhythm disorders for me. On the one hand, one had to really understand the ECG and how it came about here, and on the other hand, these were all patients in whom one could make a wrong diagnosis or take the wrong measures and thus make things worse (the classic: Isoptin in an unrecognized WPW syndrome). Since one cannot, of course, choose the call-outs and patients in an emergency service, I had, according to my personal motto "face your fears", at some point studied all the common Lown classifications and other rhythm classifications as well as the available, mostly Greek-sounding antiarrhythmics intensively and differentiated. So I felt well prepared and hoped for an early call-out!

This call-out came about two months later and manifested itself in the form of an attractive 24-year-old student in her equally attractive 4-woman flat share. I knew that I could now reap the rewards for my intensive preparation and efforts and appear competent and justified. The student reported that she had been feeling an intense heart palpitation for about an hour, which had suddenly started. She denied any pain or shortness of breath. Since she actually wanted to go to sports

J. Koppenberg (✉)
Department of Anesthesiology, Pain Therapy and Emergency Medicine,
OSPIDAL – Center da sandà Engiadina Bassa, Scuol, Switzerland
e-mail: Joachim.Koppenberg@cseb.ch

with her friends, a friend had called the emergency services to ask whether the heart problems could be serious, which is why we were alarmed. The blood pressure was 115/65 mmHg, peripheral oxygen saturation was 99% and the 3-channel ECG (at that time there were no 12-channel ECGs on the ambulance) showed a regular, narrow and tachycardic rhythm with a frequency of 148/min. While I tried to insert a venous access in rather difficult vein conditions, the further past medical history did not reveal any special findings: Such an episode had never occurred before, no relevant previous illnesses, no allergies, no regular medication, non-smoker, no and especially no recent drug use, no current psychological emergency situation, no fever, no infection, no pain—in short, everything bland. So a young, healthy student with palpitations for an hour with a regular narrow complex tachycardia. But she was fortunately helped—after all, I had learned my EKG rhythm lessons and she was lucky that I was on duty today! The patient probably saw this after the second attempt at a venous access at this point. After the venous access was finally placed with some effort, I first explained to her and the interested bystanders in detail and with as many important sounding foreign terms as possible that the first step in therapy according to the algorithm was the Valsalva maneuvers. The present ladies were initially very impressed, but the mood tipped more towards the ridiculous when my complex representation resulted in successive unsuccessful massage of the neck, closed eyes, whistling and drinking of cold water. I felt how my competence was increasingly called into question, although I was really extremely well prepared! But of course it wasn't over with the medical art yet—according to the algorithm, the medicinal measures were now used. I explained to the audience that I would now use a very short-acting medication (adenosine) to stop the heart for a short time—this could also cause a short feeling of tightness in the patient's chest. But the patient really shouldn't worry, because the heart "jumps" again and again on its own and I would rather not speak of a short "asystole", but rather of a "pre-systolic pause"—this would sound much more hopeful! In addition, we of course also had all the equipment for necessary advanced resuscitation measures including artificial ventilation and defibrillation—so nothing could go wrong. The cheerfulness in the room disappeared abruptly and I could be sure of the respect of the audience again. After I had discussed the procedure with the paramedics and checked all the equipment again for their functioning, I therefore injected 6 mg adenosine intravenously in a bolus and immediately flushed with the infusion. The EKG rhythm became slower and slower and, as expected, the patient briefly rolled her eyes and then, yes, then the heart jumped back into a sinus rhythm with a frequency of 78/min. I had done it! There was great relief among all those involved in the room and so there was no objection that we would take the stable patient to the nearby emergency room of the city hospital for further clarification. During the journey, the patient thanked me several times for the successful treatment.

When I arrived at the hospital, I proudly demanded the on-call cardiologist for the handover, after all, I also wanted to get the knight's accolade from the clinician. When he appeared reluctantly and I told him the course and of my successful treatment, he remained silent until the end. When I was done with my detailed and algorithm-based explanations and waiting for the hymn of praise for the cured patient who was admitted to the emergency room, he looked long at the 12-channel ECG that was just being written in the emergency room and then turned to me: "And what did the patient have?" I am confused and answer: "A regular, narrow complex tachycardia—I said that already." "Yes, but what was the cause? The current 12-channel ECG is completely unimpressive—did you write a 12-channel ECG before the measures to find the cause?" Now I realized that the man had no idea of pre-hospital emergency medicine! "As you should know, we don't have a 12-channel ECG on the ambulance," I replied already somewhat unfriendly. "So, so" said the cardiologist in a paternal tone "then you can just as well take the patient home again and we all wait until she has such an event again and then hopefully an emergency physician is called who either doesn't know what to do in such a case or knows it very well, but realizes that you don't need to treat and endanger a stable patient unnecessarily in the living room and thus screw up our diagnostics at the same time! Have a nice day."—and he was gone. I stood there like a drowned poodle and couldn't understand what he wanted to say to me at all. Fortunately, an internal medicine emergency room resident took pity on me and took over the patient, who in turn did not fail to thank me again for the extremely competent help.

Discussion
It really took me a few days and several conversations to slowly admit to myself how right the cardiologist was. But I only meant well—but "well-intentioned" is not good enough for our patients. First of all, it is certainly still not reprehensible to deal with the things one is afraid of ("face your fears") or to acquire in-depth knowledge, as in this specific case with regard to ECG rhythm disorders and their therapy. However, in emergency medicine, one must not automatically use what has been learned everywhere and at all times, but always take into account the external circumstances and use the knowledge accordingly differentiated. First of all, I should have clearly stated from the outset that the student was always cardiopulmonary stable and at no time vital and thus not necessarily in need of treatment in her apartment. This is what the guidelines of the American Heart Association and the European Resuscitation Council agree on for this purpose, that in the case of stable narrow complex tachycardias, a 12-channel ECG should be made first for the purpose of diagnosis, which we did not have at that time on the ambulance or physician-manned ambulance. After that, one should weigh up very well whether one has to initiate a therapy at all, since each of them can also act proarrhythmically and clinically worsen the previously stable situation. Therefore, consultation of an expert is recommended if possible—in our case the cardiologist in the emergency room. Despite the knowledge of what would actually be done, I should have simply monitored the patient, inserted an intravenous access and brought her to the next

emergency room—no more, but also no less. Although it is certainly more difficult to omit something that one knows or masters than if one has great respect for it. So it was great luck that the medication therapy initiated in a spectacular way in the living room was successful and the patient was not put into an unnecessary extreme situation or endangered by my "too much knowledge".

Of course, one could argue whether one could not try the "harmless" vagus or Valsalva maneuvers in the apartment nevertheless. Here the second legitimate criticism of the cardiologist comes into play: Even if these maneuvers are successful in up to 25%, we would still not know what was the cause of the rhythm disorders (differential diagnosis in this case: sinus tachycardia, AV node reentry tachycardia, atrioventricular reentry tachycardias due to WPW syndrome, atrial flutter with regular AV conduction, focal atrial tachycardia) and whether the patient needed further clarification or therapy before the therapy. Therefore, one should only initiate the therapy in stable patients if one has a diagnosis or has written a 12-channel ECG for later evaluation. In addition, a 12-channel ECG must be connected during the therapy measures, as some rhythm disorders can only be safely identified in the phase of unmasking. Of course, this procedure is only recommended for cardiopulmonary stable patients. If the patient is or becomes unstable, a medical or electrical therapy (cardioversion) must be initiated immediately according to guidelines. But then it is the case that the patient or his condition forces us to an immediate therapy. The decisive factor is therefore that we always treat the patients as a whole and never just an atypical ECG picture, even if we can interpret it correctly!

33.1 Conclusion

This case led me for the first time in my career as an emergency physician to the realization that even the renunciation of treatment in the interest of the patient can be right and often "less is more". Our performance is not always measured by the number of actions. This is—to be honest—not easy to control, because we are usually (especially emergency) medicine strong action- and impulse-triggered and the perceived quality of our work often correlates with the number of measures taken. But we must never only treat individual values or ECG images, but always look at and treat our patients as a whole. And this even when a much younger colleague in the emergency room indirectly suggests ignorance to us later, because we would have treated this obvious symptom long ago! Finally, it should be emphasized once again that it is not bad to deal intensively with the things that scare us, according to the motto "face your fears".

Further Reading

1. Deakin CD, Nolan JP, Soar J et al (2010) Advanced life support for adults. Notfall Rettungsmed 13:559–620
2. Neumar RW, Otto CW, Link MS et al (2010) Part 8: adult advanced cardiovascular life support. Circulation 11(suppl 3):729–767
3. Soar J, Böttiger BW, Carli P, Couper K, Deakin CD, Djärv T, Lott C, Olasveengen T, Paal P, Pellis T, Perkins GD, Sandroni C, Nolan JP. European Resuscitation Council Guidelines 2021: Adult advanced life support. Resuscitation. 2021 Apr; 161:115–151. https://doi.org/10.1016/j.resuscitation.2021.02.010. Epub 2021 Mar 24. Erratum in: Resuscitation. 2021 Oct; 167:105–106. PMID: 33773825.

Fall While Downhill Mountainbiking

Martin Messelken

▶ In this case, it is about a call to an outdoor application and the associated adverse conditions found there, which are partly compensated by personal commitment and improvisation of the respective teams, in order to achieve a good result for the patients

The emergency call for the EMS helicopter is: "Mountain biker fallen in forest; exact coordinates still to be determined". Just under 2 min later, the EMS helicopter is in the air for a 12-minute approach. The visibility on this late summer morning is not restricted. The target area turns out to be a densely wooded slope of a contiguous forest, no signals or people in need of help can be seen. After the 3rd flyover, the pilot discovers a sight-seeing platform on the slope that fits the specified target location precisely from the control center. "Can you jump down if I only land with a skid on the railing of the sight-seeing platform?" asks the pilot. I agree and get ready to exit with the large emergency backpack. Much faster than I thought, I am alone on the platform and my EMS helicopter has flown away without the option to land—so I am alone, without a radio and cut off from communication, as there is no mobile phone signal at all. Fortunately, a cyclist emerges from the forest and leads me to his injured comrade. The 25-year-old cyclist had underestimated a jump hill while riding downhill, lost control of his mountain bike and crashed heavily on his buttocks and back; but he was conscious all the time. Except for painful bruises, nothing serious was found during the cranio-caudal body check (ABCDE). I put on a neck brace, prepared an infusion, injected 0.1 mg fentanyl intravenously and was glad when two paramedics arrived a few minutes later—their ambulance is 500 m (547 yards) away on a forest path. With their

M. Messelken (✉)
Bad Boll, Germany
e-mail: m.messelken@gmail.com

V. Wenzel (ed.), *Case Studies in Emergency Medicine*,
https://doi.org/10.1007/978-3-662-67249-5_34

radio we can contact the EMS helicopter; due to the circumstances of the accident, we decide to transport the patient to the ambulance with a Spineboard via the narrow forest path. The four of us should be able to do that. When I look at the unlucky bike, I notice a Garmin outdoor navigation device on its handlebars and ask: "Why didn't you give us the GPS coordinates of the accident site? You can read them there. We could have found you faster." "Actually, that's right," was the answer, "but how does that work?" The ambulance transports us with the patient to the EMS helicopter landing site in an industrial area; there we unload the injured and fly to the next trauma surgery emergency room. This is routine.

Discussion

After this call, there was, of course, a lot to discuss. This was mainly due to the explicit absence of a preparing and the abrupt team separation. This was associated with a critical restriction of communication means and therapy options. Fortunately, this did not turn out to be a specific disadvantage, as our patient was not seriously injured—but it could have been quite different. As a consequence of this incident, a few days later a small, easy-to-handle backpack for mobile first aid was equipped and carried along to begin initial cardiorespiratory therapy and monitoring in such cases with a self-inflating ventilation bag, intubation material, venous access and infusion, pulse oximeter and blood pressure measurement (anesthetics are always carried along personally anyway) .

Mountain bikers often have accidents in inaccessible terrain due to self-induced falls. The accident risks are comparable to those of alpine skiing [1]. The timely alarm of the EMS, the determination and reaching of the accident site often take place under non-regular conditions—all deviations are due to an Outdoorsituation and life-threatening is not necessarily compatible. Nevertheless, fatal accidents are rather rare. The outdoor navigation wearables carried along in many cases provide GPS coordinates at the touch of a button. If the mountain bikers had familiarized themselves with the function before and transmit this data to the EMS control center, valuable time can be saved in the search for the intervention site. This can be life-saving in particular if hypothermia sets in and a search for the possibly single-track victim at night is difficult and time-consuming. In some communities, such as Innsbruck, Austria, the EMS control center even provides a free app for smartphones with which you can extremely accurately inform the rescue workers of your own location after turning on the GPS function.

34.1   Conclusion

The description of my unforgettable emergency interventions represents only a small part of the spectrum of an emergency physician active for over 3 decades [2]. With a view to the limited treatment options of earlier years, special attention is paid to structural weaknesses which were partly compensated by the personal commitment and improvisation of the respective teams in order to achieve a good result for the patients. The medical and operational documentation in connection with intensive data analysis has been further developed since then and led, via applied quality management, to measurable improvement of the result quality in many cases [3]. The rapidly developing information technology was a constant companion—so at the beginning of my work as an emergency physician we did not even have a pulse oximeter and 30 years later GPS-supported interventions were possible.

References

1. Armold M (2005) Mountainbiken. Orthopade 5:405–410
2. Bernhard M et al (2006) Spectrum of patients in prehospital emergency services. What has changed over the last 20 years? Anaesthesist 55(11):1157–1165
3. Messelken M et al (2010) The quality of emergency medical care in Baden-Wurttemberg (Germany): four years in focus. Dtsch Arztebl Int 107(30):523–530

Serious Head Injury

35

Peter Hilbert-Carius

▶ What to do when several problems have to be solved at the same time? Where to start, where to continue, where to stop? In this case, many problems come together that the rescue and emergency room team have to master.

The emergency room team of a regional trauma center is informed by the EMS control center that a severe open head trauma will arrive in about 10 min. In addition, it is transmitted that the patient is being ventilated. A short time later, about 2 min before the patient arrives, the EMS control center receives another information that the patient is now undergoing cardiopulmonary resuscitation (CPR) and will reach the hospital within a few minutes. Shortly thereafter, the patient arrives in an ambulance with an emergency physician and is received by the emergency room team at the ambulance. CPR of a patient with asystole is ongoing. The airway is secured with a laryngeal mask, but no thoracic excursions are visible during CPR during ventilation; an end-expiratory CO_2 measurement is not connected. The patient is then transported to the emergency room with ongoing CPR. As part of a first quick Primary Survey according to ATLS®, the following problems quickly become apparent:

- A (Airway)—secured by means of a laryngeal mask, but no ventilation is possible;
- B (Breathing)—no ventilation of the lungs on both sides;
- C (Circulation)— circulatory arrest with asystole;
- D (Disability)—GCS 3, pupils on both sides wide without light reaction;

P. Hilbert-Carius (✉)
Department of Anesthesiology, Intensive Care, and Emergency Medicine,
BG Trauma Hospital Bergmannstrost, Halle / Saale, Germany
e-mail: Dr.PeterHilbert@web.de

© The Author(s), under exclusive license to Springer-Verlag GmbH, DE, part of Springer Nature 2023
V. Wenzel (ed.), *Case Studies in Emergency Medicine*,
https://doi.org/10.1007/978-3-662-67249-5_35

- E (Exposure/Environment)—ongoing CPR, right frontal head injury, no other signs of injury.

There are therefore several serious problems, so that first an attempt is made to solve the problem with the highest priority, the A-problem. For this purpose, the laryngeal mask is removed and the patient is intubated with direct laryngoscopy, which succeeds without problems on the first attempt. After intubation, the tube position is checked by auscultation and equal-sided respiratory sounds and parallel good visible thoracic excursion as well as expiratory CO_2 of 18 mmHg is recorded during ongoing CPR. It has thus been possible to solve the existing A and B problems, but circulatory arrest is still present. With continuation of CPR and after the second injection of 1 mg epinephrine intravenously, ventricular action is first seen on the ECG, which converts to sinus rhythm after a short time. The end-expiratory CO_2 rises to values of 80 mmHg and a carotid pulse is palpable. With a continuation of a low-dose catecholamine therapy with 0.01 µg/kg/min norepinephrine, circulation remains stable in the further course. Then a re-evaluation of the condition is carried out with the following result:

- A – intubated ventilated, correct tube position;
- B – lungs ventilated on both sides, peripheral oxygen saturation of 100% with FiO_2 of 1.0;
- C – circulation stable with low noradrenaline requirement (blood pressure 115/85 mmHg, heart rate 106/min);
- D – GCS 3, pupils still dilated on both sides without light reaction;
- E – known head injury.

In the blood gas analysis, severe combined acidosis with pronounced respiratory and only minor metabolic component is shown, which is slowly compensated by adjustment of ventilation. In the whole-body CT, in addition to the known head injury, no further injuries are visible. The following past medical history of the accident is to be learned from the emergency physician: The patient was an inmate of a penal institution and a known epileptic. He probably had another attack today and fallen in the process, injuring his head. When the emergency physician arrived, the patient was somnolent and had a Glasgow Coma Scale of 8. Due to the suspected head injury and the Glasgow Coma Scale of 8, an indication for intubation was made. After induction of anesthesia, intubation was not possible in several attempts, so that a laryngeal mask was used as an alternative strategy. With this, the patient's ventilation was initially possible and, under the suspicion of a severe open head injury, transport to a regional trauma center was initiated. On the way there, ventilation problems occurred at first and, in the further course, cardiac arrest with the need for resuscitation. After completion of the diagnosis and treatment of the patient with all necessary invasive lines, he is transferred to the intensive care unit, treated there for 24 h by means of hypothermia and then slowly rewarmed. Despite these measures, the patient only wakes up very delayed and is transferred to a rehabilitation hospital after 3 weeks with a pronounced neurological damage.

Discussion

The case demonstrates how a chain of unfortunate circumstances and decisions can lead to deleterious consequences that would most likely have been completely avoidable. First, the patient, known to be an epileptic, has a seizure and falls. This is not entirely atypical, and that one might sustain a head injury in such a fall does not seem so unusual. The postictal somnolence that often follows most seizures, which can vary greatly in length and intensity, is then of course difficult to interpret. The somnolence of the patient was probably more likely seen by the emergency physician as a result of the supposed head trauma and the possibility of a postictal state considered less likely. Consequently, the decision to intubate, which should be done according to various guidelines in the event of a head trauma with a Glasgow Coma Scale of ≤ 8 [1, 2], was the logical consequence. Unfortunately, conventional intubation also failed outside of the hospital in several attempts, so that a laryngeal mask was used. This strategy was initially also successful and the patient could be ventilated and oxygenated with the laryngeal mask. The chosen approach after failed intubation to switch to a supraglottic airway such as the laryngeal mask is in line with current recommendations for prehospital airway management [3] and proved to be initially practicable. Regardless of the initial successful use of the laryngeal mask, problems can also occur when using supraglottic airway devices. Some of the most important problems are only mentioned here by way of example: airway obstruction by dislocation, aspiration, gastric distension, hypoventilation, injuries (bleeding, tongue swelling), and unnoticed dislocation. An interesting case series of possible problems with the supraglottic airway alternative laryngeal tube was described by Bernhard et al. in a publication that can only be recommended to the interested reader [4].

Apparently, a problem occurred during transport that made ventilation more difficult and eventually impossible. Since this problem was obviously not recognized or eliminated, there was pronounced hypoventilation and hypoxia with subsequent cardiac arrest in the further course of the transport. The fact that a $paCO_2$ of 80 mmHg (10.6 kPa) was present in the blood gas analysis taken shortly after elimination of this problem clearly demonstrates the hypoventilation. Ultimately, problems with ventilation led to the catastrophic outcome of this case. Therefore, clinical control (inspection, percussion, auscultation), pulse oximetry and capnometry/-graphy as well as the control of volumes and airway pressures must be demanded as EMS basic measures for monitoring ventilation. The fact that diagnostics, with the exception of the already pre-hospital visible head injury, did not reveal any trauma consequences makes the case even more tragic, since ultimately misinterpretation of a postictal drowsy state after seizure was responsible for the subsequent events. Ultimately, however, misinterpretation could have remained without negative consequences for the patient if the problems that had occurred in the pre-hospital course had been recognized and treated adequately as part of airway management and mechanical ventilation. Therefore, it can only be appealed again and again that every colleague working in emergency and intensive medicine intensively deals with the topic airway management and ventilation and anticipates possible problems in advance [5].

35.1 Conclusion

An important aspect that should be emphasized is the fact that after the supposed solution of a problem (here securing of the airway), one must re-evaluate in the further course whether the problem has really been solved or remains and whether perhaps a new problem has arisen. This re-evaluation is a basic pillar of ATLS® (Advanced Trauma Life Support) and PHTLS® (Prehospital Trauma Life Support), which in the context of trauma care suggest a priority-oriented approach according to the A, B, C, D, E scheme [6, 7]. If there are several problems at the same time (see above), the one with the highest priority, in our case the A (Airway) problem, is solved before the other problems are addressed. In line with the principle "Treat first what kills first". Under early consideration of the basics and principles of ATLS®/PHTLS®, which are actually nothing more than well-known basics of emergency medicine, a re-evaluation of supposedly solved problems in the described case would have quickly made it clear that the unsolved A-problem ultimately led to the need for resuscitation and not the "open head injury".

References

1. Deutsche Gesellschaft für Unfallchirurgie e. V. (DGU) (2011) Polytrauma/Schwerverletzten-Behandlung. AWMF-Register Nr. 012/019 Klasse: S3
2. Donaubauer B, Fakler J, Gries A, Kaisers UX, Josten C, Bernhard M (2014) Interdisciplinary management of trauma patients: update 3 years after implementation of the S3 guidelines on treatment of patients with severe and multiple injuries. Anaesthesist 63:852–864
3. Timmermann A, Byhahn C, Wenzel V et al (2012) Handlungsempfehlung für das präklinische Atemwegsmanagement. Für Notärzte und Rettungsdienstpersonal. Anästh Intensivmed 53:294–308
4. Bernhard M, Beres W, Timmermann A et al (2014) Prehospital airway management using the laryngeal tube: an emergency department point of view. Anaesthesist 63:589–596
5. Bernhard M, Bein B, Böttiger BW, Bohn A, Fischer M, Gräsner JT, Hinkelbein J, Kill C, Lott C, Popp E, Roessler M, Schaumberg A, Wenzel V, Hossfeld B (2015) Handlungsempfehlung zur prähospitalen Notfallnarkose beim Erwachsenen. Anästh Intensivmed 56:317–335
6. Helm M, Kulla M, Lampl L (2007) Advanced trauma life support(R): a training concept also for Europe. Anaesthesist 56:1142–1146
7. Thies KC, Nagele P (2007) Advanced trauma life support(R) – a standard of care for Germany?: no substantial improvement of care can be expected. Anaesthesist 56:1147–1154

A Nearly Deadly Tea

Hermann Brugger

▶ Intoxications present the emergency medical team with a difficult task: is the intoxication source known? And if so, is there an antidote? In this case, it is also about the resource question and how to act as effectively as possible with the few options that are available.

Half of the Pustertal valley in South Tyrol, Italy lives of one ski mountain. The Kronplatz, centrally located between primeval rock and the Dolomites, stretches its white tentacles in all directions in winter. In the north and east they reach to Bruneck and Olang, in the south to the municipality of Enneberg with the village of St. Vigil. In this region, new lifts, hotels, guesthouses and whole new settlements sprang up. During the ski season, all houses are booked up, the skiers are during the day on the mountain and in the evening in restaurants and nightclubs. High season is also for the EMS, which shuttle 24 h a day between the holiday resorts and the district hospital Bruneck.

In the off-season spring and autumn, however, there is lonely peace here. This affects the restaurants and hotels, but also brings us emergency physicians a breather; the absolute low point of the statistics is the month of November. The ski season has not yet begun and hoteliers and restaurant operators are lying on the beaches in the south or in the mud of the Abano thermal baths; only a few remain. So it is quite possible that you can sleep through the night in the emergency service. Quite different on this Monday. At 2:00 am the alarm rings. Medical emergency, deployment location in a small village. We start in the physician-manned ambulance, inquire on the way for further details and learn that the local EMS is already on site with an ambulance with a driver and paramedic and has found 3

H. Brugger (✉)
EURAC Research, Bozen, Italy, Institute of Mountain Emergency Medicine, Bozen, Italy
e-mail: hermann.brugger@eurac.edu

V. Wenzel (ed.), *Case Studies in Emergency Medicine*,
https://doi.org/10.1007/978-3-662-67249-5_36

unconscious youths in a new settlement. According to the information of the first arriving paramedics, all 3 affected persons have spontaneous respiration. I give the first instructions over the radio: stable side-lying, observation, exploration of the environment. After about 30 min drive through the narrow valley we arrive. The settlement, indeed the whole village is deserted, light is only visible in the affected apartment. When I enter this with my paramedic, the following picture presents itself: 2 male youths lie motionless in the kitchen, another female person in the living room, all on the floor, brought into stable side-lying by the local paramedics. At the first vital check I can determine a carotid pulse and spontaneous respiration in all, but only the girl reacts specifically to pain stimuli, makes incomprehensible sounds and opens her eyes on request (Glasgow Coma Scale 11). The two boys show an uncoordinated pain response and open their eyes to pain stimuli, but one of the two has no verbal response (Glasgow Coma Scale 9 and 6), while he only breathes flat and irregularly. Systolic blood pressure is around 100 mmHg in all, oxygen saturation is 97% in the girl, 88 and 90% in the boys. In all of them we notice wide light-fixed pupils.

Now several questions arise: can and should I secure the airways of these unconscious young patients for transport in several vehicles? A phone call to the EMS dispatch center makes it clear that a second emergency physician is not available; per EMS vehicle, only one patient can be transported lying down. If I intubate 2 patients, the paramedic in the EMS vehicle would have to take care of an intubated patient alone, which I do not want to burden them with. An intubation and mechanical ventilation of all 3 patients is therefore not an option, not only because of the lack of personnel, but also because of the lack of a additional ventilators. I therefore request another ambulance with oxygen and monitor.

The second question is at least as urgent as the first: what happened that 3 young people are suddenly deeply unconscious? None of them smells of alcohol, a metabolic cause is unlikely in view of the simultaneous onset of unconsciousness, the blood sugar test is normal in all of them, there is no indication of a gas leak such as carbon monoxide. An external agent is more than likely and the wide pupils make us think of an intoxication. I first decide to anesthetize the worst of the 3 young people with a muscle relaxant and propofol with the assistance of my experienced paramedic, intubate and mechanically ventilate him. All 3 young people are monitored and provided with an intravenous access. I send my paramedic to the second boy with the request to continuously observe breathing, pulse and oxygen saturation and to immediately notify me of any deterioration. I send another paramedic to the girl for monitoring. At the same time, I ask the two paramedics of the ambulance to search the apartment for drugs, suspicious food or medication residues and to find possible witnesses in the neighborhood who may have observed something. However, the search for suspicious substances remains unsuccessful. After a while, one of the two paramedics comes back with a housemate who has remained indifferent and unnoticed in his apartment so far and says: "I only know one of the two boys; the parents are on vacation and, as far as I know, unreachable, I don't know the other two." However, he draws our attention to the fact that the trio has met here several times. He has observed that they have been busy with flowers on the balcony several times. Now we only notice that there is an empty teapot and half-full cups on the kitchen table. One of the paramedics goes to the balcony and immediately comes back with a funnel-shaped light yellow flower and the triumphant exclamation: "Angel trumpet!" Now we also notice leaf residues on the kitchen table. Maybe there is a plant poisoning? I know that angel trumpets are poisonous, but I don't know the effect. Well, I think, we know what it is most likely, now we can prepare for transport. After a short discussion with the paramedics and the driver of the physician-manned ambulance, we decide to divide the patients into 3 vehicles and now drive in convoy to the hospital: the intubated patient in the physician-manned ambulance, the second boy in the ambulance and the girl in the other ambulance, all with monitoring and oxygen. While the girl is somnolent and largely stable, the non-intubated boy remains unconscious. Then I call the Poison Control Center in Vienna, Austria and inquire about the effects of angel trumpets and an antidote; they explain to me: "Angel trumpets are highly poisonous and have an atropine-like effect; the antidote is physostigmine intravenously 1–2 mg at 10 min intervals." Unfortunately, I can't find anything like that in the ambulance.

During the ride, my patient remains circulatory stable and I am in constant radio contact with the other two EMS vehicles; I report our patients to the hospital and request the antidote for the emergency room. Shortly after arrival, we inject all 3 patients with 1 mg of physostigmine in a short infusion and can see the condition improve after a few minutes. The girl becomes responsive, and after repeating the dose, the second boy's condition also normalizes. The intubated patient remains sedated and can be extubated the following day. 3 days later, all have left the hospital.

Discussion
Poisonings from angel's trumpets primarily affect children and adolescents for various reasons [1]. With small children, it can happen due to the carelessness of the parents if leaves or flowers are taken into the mouth and chewed. Adolescents, on the other hand, usually know about the intoxicating effect and take plant parts intentionally; mostly in the form of extracts as tea, by chewing plant parts, or smoking dried leaves [2]. Extracts of the angel's trumpet are also popular as intoxicants among indigenous peoples of South America. In Europe, the angel's trumpet (Brugmansia) is an ornamental plant that is kept in gardens or as a potted plant. All plant parts contain high concentrations (up to 0.5%) of the poisonous alkaloids hyoscyamine and scopolamine, whose atropine-like effects are known: 1–2 h after ingestion, there is a dose-dependent euphoric mood, excitement, hallucinations, mydriasis, clouding of consciousness, coma, circulatory insufficiency, and in rare cases, circulatory failure. Aggressive actions have also been described [3], but also long-lasting flashbacks with hallucinations. The angel's trumpet is a highly toxic plant with the highest natural content of alkaloids, where

the concentration in the plant parts is different and unpredictable—50 mg can already be fatal. Therefore, uncontrolled ingestion or intake is strongly discouraged; intravenous injection of a potent cholinergic such as physostigmine is recommended as an antidote.

The actual problem of this intervention was less the emergency medical treatment of intoxication than the absolute scarcity of resources in a remote valley. Fortunately, the maximum effect of the toxin had already been reached in all 3 patients when our EMS team arrived, so that no deterioration occurred during transport. Otherwise, ventilation and, in the worst case, cardiopulmonary resuscitation of several people would have been inevitable. I do not want to imagine what this would have meant in practice; most likely it would have led to an EMS disaster, since both the personnel and the equipment would have been lacking to treat and monitor several intubation-dependent patients. First of all, it becomes evident here how difficult the management of several intubation-dependent patients can be in remote regions with long travel times, especially if the situation is not evident from the beginning, but only on site and the re-alarm of additional personnel and equipment becomes the main problem. In our case, there was no background service available; but even if that had been the case, the second physician would have reached us in 30–40 min.

The following summer I returned by car from a mountain tour in the Dolomites; I saw a man by the roadside who was hitchhiking home. I picked up the hitchhiker, noticed that he looked familiar to me and asked him where he was going—in fact he wanted to go to the village where I had treated the 3. Slowly it dawned on me that he might be the intubated boy. I asked in passing if he had been in hospital last winter? He said spontaneously: "Yes, with a severe intoxication! I tell you—that was terrible, I still have nightmares and I would not wish it on anyone … ". I said nothing and did not reveal that I was the emergency physician.

36.1 Conclusion

In patients with suspicious behavior or impaired consciousness up to coma, one should not forget the possibility of plant poisoning. Contacting a poison center can speed up the therapeutic effect, but of course it is of no use if the antidote is not carried in the EMS or the intoxication is not recognized as such. Even in non-traumatic events, it can happen that intubation-dependent patients become multiple at the same time; in rural regions with long travel times, this can turn into an event that is hardly manageable. Therefore, a background service with a second physician available is particularly important.

References

1. Francis PD, Clarke CF (1999) Angel trumpet lily poisoning in five adolescents: clinical findings and management. J Paediatr Child Health 35(1):93–95
2. Niess C, Schnabel A, Kauert G (1999) Angel trumpet: a poisonous garden plant as a new addictive drug? Dtsch Med Wochenschr 124(48):1444–1447
3. Marneros A, Gutmann P, Uhlmann F (2006) Self-amputation of penis and tongue after use of Angel's Trumpet. Eur Arch Psychiatry Clin Neurosci 256(7):458–459

Abandoned Newborn

Peer G. Knacke

▶ What if the patient who needs emergency care is not only a few days old, but only a few hours old? What aspects of this treatment make it particularly necessary for the rescue workers to think about? The present case is very illustrative of this special situation.

Our EMS helicopter is the large Bell 212 with two rotor blades and the therefore far audible "flapp-flapp", which many people call the "sound of rescue". It is a wintery cold, but sunny November day when we are alerted by the EMS control center. A physician-manned ambulance and an ambulance are already on site; as an additional remark it is said that the EMS helicopter should come without a stretcher. We discuss in the team why this might be necessary. From a perforation injury with a large object in our rural catchment area to the avoidance of a re-positioning or a very, very obese patient, much is considered. But everything remains uncertain. Further information about the mission is also not available via radio in busy radio traffic the EMS control center. During the landing approach, the physician-manned ambulance as well as 2 ambulances are visible on the road, but no accident vehicle is to be seen. Near the vehicles we land, I take our special equipment of the EMS helicopter as usual and we are curious what awaits us.

Then we are really surprised: In the ambulance, in addition to the first arrived physician and two EMS assistants, an incubator is to be seen in which a newborn lies and is ventilated with bag-mask ventilation. Immediately our EMS helicopter technical crew member assistant is asked to fetch the children's emergency case. We did not expect that at all! The physician describes that the infant had

P. G. Knacke (✉)
Department of Anesthesiology and Emergency Medicine, AMEOS Hospitals Ostholstein, Eutin, Germany
e-mail: p.knacke@t-online.de

V. Wenzel (ed.), *Case Studies in Emergency Medicine*,
https://doi.org/10.1007/978-3-662-67249-5_37

been found naked about 90 min earlier in a garbage can at an outside temperature of $-4\,°C$ (24.8 °F). The incubator had then been requested and brought to the scene of the accident with the second ambulance; the request of our EMS helicopter without stretcher had been made so that the incubator fits well into the EMS helicopter. Our little patient is a hypotrophic appearing, mature newborn boy. The examination shows clearly disturbed vital functions. Despite bag-mask ventilation with oxygen and reservoir bag, there is a significant cyanosis. The boy is completely limp, spontaneous respiration is not detectable, nor is a pulse palpable with an EKG heart rate of 30/min. The pupils are dilated on both sides and without light reaction, the already determined blood sugar is at 100 mg/dl. A measurement of body temperature is not possible because a thermometer with a measuring possibility in the hypothermic range does not belong to the EMS equipment at the time of the mission.

I intubate the boy with a Glasgow Coma Scale of 3 orotracheally without problems with a tube (ID 2.5) at an insertion depth of 10 cm and use the breathing apparatus of the incubator (Babylog®) known to me from pediatric training for ventilation (FiO$_2$ 1.0; respiratory rate 35, maximum ventilation pressure 20 mbar). With this, the child becomes pinker and the heart rate rises to 45/min. Then a peripheral venous access is established on the back of the hand, which fortunately succeeds on the first attempt. 30 µg adrenaline and two fractionated doses of 30 µg atropine are injected via this access. With still no palpable pulse, we infuse 10 ml HAES 6% and an infusion of 40 ml glucose 5% with 10 ml NaCl 0.9% with 20 ml/h via a syringe pump. Since there is still no pulse palpable, we decide to transport the already ventilated child under thoracic compressions ground-based to a hospital of maximum care with pediatric cardiac surgery and thus the possibility of extracorporeal warming via a heart-lung machine. The pre-notification "newborn resuscitation in hypothermia" is made via the EMS control center, the estimated transport time is 20 min. With the necessary repositioning and also during ongoing cardiopulmonary resuscitation, the air transport proposed by the first arriving doctor offers no advantages. The transport takes place without problems. The transfer takes place according to the specification of the hospital directly on the pediatric intensive care unit. There the rectal temperature measurement is 22 °C (71.6 °F). The thoracic compressions are discontinued and the rewarming is slowly carried out in the incubator under constant defibrillation readiness. Extracorporeal circulation is not used for rewarming; the rewarming succeeds in the incubator without problems. The mother immediately placed the child in the trash can after the birth; therefore, the boy is given up for adoption. In the clinical follow-up examinations, no neurological abnormalities can be detected. Meanwhile, the boy lives healthy with his adoptive parents.

Discussion

The provision of deep hypothermic newborns is an absolute rarity in emergency medical services and requires the team special skills and knowledge. So the skills of endotracheal intubation, the establishment of venous accesses and the administration of intraosseous cannulas can be learned only by clinical experience as part of internships and training courses. In addition, there are uncertainties and dangerous miscalculations in the dosing of emergency drugs, as one can easily miscalculate by a factor of 10 when calculating a dilution. To prevent these problems, it is absolutely recommended to carry dosage aids for pediatric emergencies in every pediatric emergency kit [1]. The resuscitation recommendations for newborns from 2021 are to breathe with room air first in the event of apnea and a heart rate <100/min with a free airway, and to additionally perform chest compressions over the lower third of the sternum if the heart rate is below 60/min and the lungs are safely ventilated. Chest compressions and ventilation should be in a ratio of 3:1 (compression frequency 120 per minute). If, despite effective ventilation, there is no satisfactory increase in the pre-ductal pulse oximetry-measured oxygen saturation, the oxygen concentration should be increased [7]. In our case, we first performed chest compressions in addition to the primary securing of ventilation in the event of persistent low heart rate and undetectable pulse. At the time of deployment, unfortunately, neither pre-hospital capnography nor a thermometer with the possibility of accurate measurement was available in the hypothermic range in the EMS. Both devices would have been very helpful in assessing the overall situation and are now standard equipment. The administration of HAES 6% nowadays requires a more critical indication, buffered electrolyte solutions such as Ringer's acetate solution are 1st choice [2]. To avoid further cooling, newborns should be primarily dried, wrapped in warm towels as much as possible, protected from drafts and, if necessary, kept warm at home by existing heaters.

The first stage of hypothermia is at a core body temperature of 32 to 35 °C (89.6-95 °F) (key symptom: shivering, conscious). Between 28 and 32 °C (82.4-89.6 °F) the second stage (key symptom: no shivering, consciousness impaired) is reached, the third stage is between 24 and 28 °C (75.2-82.4 °F) (key symptom: no shivering, unconscious, vital signs present) and finally the fourth stage is defined by a temperature below 24 °C (75.2 °F), in which case vital signs are usually no longer present [3]. In adults, adolescents and children, mild hypothermia initially leads to shivering, which subsides at lower temperatures; especially if hypoglycemia occurs. Therefore, the absence of shivering is considered a warning sign of deeper hypothermia. However, newborns lack the ability to produce heat through shivering. The confirmation of hypothermia should be carried out with a thermometer with a low temperature range by rectal, esophageal or tympanic measurement. In case of severe hypothermia, neither adrenaline nor other medications should be administered according to today's data until the patient has been warmed to a core body temperature of above 30 °C (86 °F). Above 30 °C (86 °F) up to a temperature of 35 °C (95 °F), injection of drugs is half as often as usual by doubling the time intervals between repeated drug administrations. Epinephrine is given intravenously and intraossarily to newborns at a dose of 10 µg/kg body weight [4].

It is not clear at which temperature and how often defibrillation should be attempted in severe hypothermia. In case of ventricular fibrillation and hypothermia, an attempt with maximum energy is allowed, with a defibrillation dose of 4 J/kg body weight in children. If ventricular fibrillation persists after three defibrillation shocks, further defibrillation attempts should only be made when a core body temperature >30 °C (86 °F) has been reached [7]. The bradycardia observed in the newborn we treated may be physiological as part of severe hypothermia; therefore, the infant was warmed in the incubator without continuing chest compressions. We used a glucose-containing solution for fluid therapy. This should be avoided in case of normoglycemia, as this can promote the development of cerebral edema. In case of suspected hypovolemia, a fluid bolus of 10–20 ml/kg body weight of isotonic saline solution is indicated. Infusion of HAES for acute volume therapy is possible under very strict indications [6].

I have never been so surprised by the EMS. But in the end everything was fine.

37.1 Conclusion

This case confirms the good prognosis (even in severe hypothermia) and that children (as well as adults) must be warmed up in order to make a meaningful decision about possible termination of resuscitation measures. Survival of severe hypothermia is quite possible, as our little patient's case demonstrates, who had no neurological abnormalities in later neuropediatric examinations. It is essential to protect infants and newborns from cooling down.

References

1. Erker CG, Santamaria M, Mollmann M (2012) Tools for drug dosing in life-threatening pediatric emergencies. Anaesthesist 61:965–970
2. Russo S, Timmermann A, Radke O, Kerren T, Brauer A (2005) Accidental hypothermia in the household environment. Importance of preclinical temperature measurement. Anaesthesist 54:1209–1214
3. Brugger H, Putzer G, Paal P (2013) Accidental hypothermia. Anaesthesist 62:624–631
4. Paal P, Brugger H, Boyd J (2013) Accidental hypothermia. N Engl J Med 368:682
5. Knacke PG, Strauß J, Gräsner JT, Saur P, Scholz J (2008) Kasuistik interaktiv: Neugeborenes mit schwerer Hypothermie Eine notärztliche Herausforderung. Anästhesiol Intensivmed Notfallmed Schmerzther 4:260–263
6. Reanimation 2021-Leitlinien kompakt. 1st edn. 2021. Deutscher Rat für Wiederbelebung

Accident While Shredding

38

Björn Hossfeld

▶ Some accidents do not immediately reveal the severity that they actually entail and only show through modern imaging what has actually happened. The present case also makes it clear that a team of rescue workers functions best when certain decisions are made by the team as a whole.

Autum fog is a nuisance for air rescue. On this day, we reported the EMS helicopter ready for duty an hour late due to morning ground fog, but now the stronger sunbeams have driven the fog away from our station and it promises to be a beautiful day. The first alarm does not take long. A neighboring EMS control center orders us to an acute eye injury. During the approach, the prudent crew of the already arrived ambulance tells us that they can hardly imagine that we will reach the scene with the EMS helicopter: there is dense fog, they cannot see the sky. We fly in a bright blue sky, but have to recognize soon that the ground fog increases under us, the closer we come to the scene. Above the scene, which is secured by GPS coordinates, it is not possible to land due to lack of visibility to the ground. However, in a few kilometers distance, the extension of the road, on which the scene is also located, appears from the fog on a hillside. Via radio, we order the ambulance to this potential landing site. Since the patient is not yet in the vehicle, a rescue assistant remains with the patient at the scene, while the other picks us up with the ambulance. A few minutes later we reach the scene and meet a municipal worker who is sitting in the lowered front loader bucket of his tractor and has a bandage over both eyes, which is bleeding on the right side.

B. Hossfeld (✉)
Department of Anesthesiology, Intensive Care, Emergency Medicine and Pain Therapy, Federal Armed Forces Hospital, Ulm, Germany
e-mail: bjoern.hossfeld@uni-ulm.de

The patient is awake and can report fluidly that he has shredded green waste from the municipality for later composting with a funnel-shaped shredder attached to the back of the tractor. While he fed more branches into the funnel, he felt a blow to his right eye and, when wiping it with his hand, found a bleed. He then turned off all the machines and informed the EMS control center with his mobile phone. The question of pain is dismissed with the remark "not so bad", he only feels a little dazed. We put the patient on the stretcher and take him to the ambulance. In order to optimize blood clotting and inspect the wound, the bandage is opened again. The upper lid of the eye is torn and shows a clear bleed; a perforation of the eyeball cannot be ruled out. No foreign body can be seen; a body check remains without further findings. While renewing the bandage, the patient asks where he is and what we are doing. Since this question is quite contrary to the previously reported course of the accident, I begin to question the patient again: in contrast to the findings a few minutes earlier, the patient is oriented to his own person, but not to time, place and course of the accident. I assume that he was hit on the head by a larger piece of wood, probably accelerated by the shredder, and caused a blunt head injury in addition to the injury to the upper eyelid. Given the more complex transport first to the EMS helicopter and then with the EMS helicopter to a suitable hospital for maximum care, I decide to induce anesthesia on site. The experienced rescue assistants first question this decision and consider anesthesia for an eye injury to be exaggerated. However, they follow my argument that the patient's neurology has deteriorated rapidly in the short time of our observation and a longer transport is pending. During an extensive preoxygenation with maximum oxygen flow and tightly fitted face mask, the further procedure is decided. Anesthesia induction and subsequent endotracheal intubation are unproblematic, as is the further transport to the emergency room of the admitting hospital. The computed tomogram made there not only astonishes the colleagues present, but also myself: Apparently, a metallic wire has penetrated deeply into the brain through the eye. In a subsequent neurosurgical procedure lasting several hours, an 11 cm long isolated copper wire can finally be removed from the front skull cavity. The eye injury is so extensive that the eye cannot be saved. 14 days after the procedure, the patient can be discharged to a neurological rehabilitation hospital with short-term memory disorders.

Discussion
The decision to administer prehospital anesthesia and the discussion with the emergency medical technicians might possibly be problematic in this case, even though the procedure turned out to be correct in retrospect. The induction of anesthesia and the resulting airway management is significantly more difficult in the prehospital setting than in the operating room, where there is always more technology, personnel, help, space, and light available than in emergency medical services [1]. Therefore, several aspects must be taken into account when making the decision to administer anesthesia in

emergency medical services: indication for anesthesia, duration and type of transport (ground-based, air-based), conditions at the scene of the accident (e.g., patient's position, lighting, space), accompanying conditions of airway management (e.g., expected intubation difficulties, possibly trapped in a car), as well as the training, experience, and routine of the EMS team [2]. The indication for prehospital intubation resulted from the patient's rapidly deteriorating neurology. This also makes it clear that the condition of a patient in emergency medicine is a dynamic process that requires constant re-evaluation in order to avoid airway disasters [3, 4] that are often initially deceptive. In a short transport to the target hospital, spontaneous breathing might also have been possible, but this was not to be expected in view of the location and weather conditions. The ambulance offers the best possible conditions for administering anesthesia in the prehospital setting because monitoring is complete and optimally positioned, and the patient is ideally positioned on the stretcher. A difficult airway was not to be expected, and the emergency physician had extensive routine in administering anesthesia and airway management.

38.1 Conclusion

Even though the emergency physician has responsibility for the mission and the patient, it is important to coordinate decisions (such as administering anesthesia) in the team and to discuss the further course of action. The assessment of the prehospital situation and the determination of suitable measures require the collection of many aspects. Together, the emergency team can use the experience of all team members. Communication is a key factor, especially in critical decisions in emergency medical services.

References

1. Bernhard M, Bein B, Böttiger BW, Bohn A, Fischer M, Gräsner JT, Hinkelbein J, Kill C, Lott C, Popp E, Roessler M, Schaumberg A, Wenzel V, Hossfeld B (2015) Recommended course of action for prehospital emergency anesthesia. Anästh Intensivmed 56:317–335
2. Timmermann A, Byhahn C, Wenzel V, Eich C, Piepho T, Bernhard M, Dörges V (2012) Recommended action for prehospital airway management. Anästh Intensivmed 53:294–308
3. Paal P, Schmid S, Herff H, von Goedecke A, Mitterlechner T, Wenzel V (2009) Excessive stomach inflation causing gut ischaemia. Resuscitation 80(1):142
4. von Goedecke A, Herff H, Paal P, Dörges V, Wenzel V (2007) Field airway management disasters. Anesth Analg 104(3):481–483

Avalanche Burial

Hermann Brugger

▶ Many factors are decisive in an avalanche accident, whether the burial can be survived and how the deployment proceeds. The present case shows which factors are decisive in the rescue mission and how dangerous such deployments can be in alpine terrain.

The three-member family from Germany is lying in front of a holiday home on the summit of an almost 2500 m (8200 feet) high ski mountain in the sun, it is March and the sun is already warming the south slopes. The slopes are less frequented, skiers and snowboarders are sitting in front of the ski huts and enjoying the warm day. A 5-year-old boy is playing a little bit apart in the snow, when he suddenly starts to cry loudly and screams: "My shovel is gone!" The father gets up from his deck chair, looks around and sees the small plastic shovel in the snow of the steep slope, which extends in front of the house towards the west into the depths and is clearly separated from the sunbathing area by a red ribbon and a large warning sign "Attention avalanche danger". He lifts the ribbon and steps into the snow; then a dull noise is heard, a piercing scream and the family father is torn into the depths by an avalanche. The mother of the little boy and other guests of the holiday home are completely horrified and call for help. When the avalanche, followed by the gaze of numerous guests, reaches the outlet at the bottom of the valley and comes to a standstill, nothing can be seen of the father of the little boy.

I am sitting in my doctor's office and taking care of the last patients when the avalanche alarm sounds. I quickly apologize to the waiting patients, exchange the white coat for the ski suit, get ski shoes, deployment backpack with skis and furs and drive to the helicopter landing pad. During the approach we receive a first

H. Brugger (✉)
EURAC Research, Institute of Mountain Emergency Medicine, Bozen, Italy
e-mail: hermann.brugger@eurac.edu

V. Wenzel (ed.), *Case Studies in Emergency Medicine*,
https://doi.org/10.1007/978-3-662-67249-5_39

layer report: "One person has fallen and is buried by an avalanche on the west slope of a mountain, further forces are being deployed". In flight we approach the slope and see a 60 cm (24 inches) high fracture below the holiday home. From there a 50 m (55 yards) wide and about 600 m (656 yards) long avalanche path leads over rocky terrain, through a narrow steep gorge, a larch forest to the flat outlet on an alpine meadow. No human being is to be seen, no trace—only huge masses of snow. At the same time we notice that only a small part of the slope has gone down and the majority of the snow masses are still hanging in the steep slope. The temperatures are high, the sun is now shining directly into the west slope and there are about 60 cm (24 inches) of fresh snow. I realize that this situation is also dangerous for us, as the slope can be unloaded at any time.

We land outside the avalanche and search the cone together as quickly as possible; after a few minutes the mountain rescuer calls me. I run to him and we see from a distance that something is moving on the snow surface: it is the head of the buried person. His body is completely buried in the snow, but the face is free and the man looks at us with big eyes, without saying anything. About 35 min have passed since the avalanche occurred.

I ask him who he is and what exactly happened, what he can explain exactly. While we dig him out of the snow in a hurry, I tell the man that he has an unimaginably large guardian angel: 600 m (656 yards) fall in an avalanche over rocks into the depths, buried by the wet snow (which is already as hard as concrete) up to the neck and almost unharmed! His answer is astonishing: "No, that's not it, I'm in good shape"! We are surprised at this carefree assessment. The patient only has a closed knee injury, a mild hypothermia (core temperature epitympanal 34 °C (93.2 °F)) and no other injuries. We stabilized the leg, hoisted the patient into the EMS helicopter and started. To fly back to the hospital, we have to overcome a mountain ridge; I take one last look back and see how the entire west slope of the mountain suddenly starts to move and a huge after-avalanche roars down the valley. It fills the entire alpine floor, including the finding site of our patient.

Discussion

The survival of an avalanche is primarily dependent on the degree of injury and burial. A burial can only be survived for more than 35 min if the avalanche victim is not fatally injured and can breathe [1]. This is the case if either the head remains unburied, as in our case (partial burial), or the whole body is buried (complete burial), but the airways are free and there is a space in front of the mouth and nose (air pocket) to breathe [2]. Otherwise, an avalanche victim will suffocate within this short period of time. With a complete burial, the probability of being alive in the avalanche is strictly time-dependent. It remains until about 20 min over 85%, drops until 35 min to 34% and after 130 min is only 7% [3]. So seen, the man had unimaginably great luck. The course of the survival probability should also be taken into account in the assessment of the danger. Up to about 35 min after the burial, it is justified to take a higher risk to rescue buried people, as the probability of finding a victim still alive is relatively high. After this time and especially after about 2 h, the chance of meeting a survivor is much lower, so that a high personal risk would not be justified.

But we rescuers were also very lucky. If we had only taken a little more time when transporting, the entire EMS helicopter team and several mountain rescuers would have been buried by the second-avalanche, but we would probably not have been as lucky as the father of the family, because the probability of being completely buried at the foot of a slope is much higher than if you are caught high up at the break-off and carried down the valley by the avalanche. We would not have been the first mountain rescuers to be buried by an avalanche: in winter 2010, two skiers were buried by an avalanche in the Bernese Uplands in Switzerland; during the rescue efforts, a second-avalanche caught 12 mountain rescuers, 4 of whom died; including the EMS helicopter physician (Berner Zeitung, 05.01.2010). In 2015, two members of an avalanche commission were caught by a slab avalanche while digging a snow profile, a standard procedure for assessing avalanche danger, and pulled into the depths, one of whom died (Tiroler Tageszeitung, 08.01.2015). At a training course of the Austrian Mountain Rescue Carinthia at Hoher Burgstall (2800 m or 9200 feet) at the end of June 2015, five participants were buried by an avalanche, two of whom died (Tiroler Tageszeitung, 22.6.2015).

A week after the avalanche, I went skiing on the same mountain myself. I pass by the holiday home and it is hardly believable: the rescued guest from our mission is already lying in the sun again and his son is playing with a shovel in the snow (I did not ask if it's the same shovel)! The man is in good condition, holds up the plaster leg and calls out to me friendly that he is looking forward to skiing again.

39.1 Conclusion

A partial burial by an avalanche is usually survived if there is no fatal trauma. With a complete burial, however, survival is strictly time-dependent and only possible with free airways and an air pocket after 35 min. Risk management by the rescue team has the highest priority in the event of an avalanche. Most avalanche accidents happen when the avalanche warning is level 3 or 4, that is, when the avalanche danger is considerable or great. The rescue teams are inevitably also exposed to this danger on the avalanche cone. In recent years, numerous mountain rescuers have died in avalanche rescue operations in Europe. All rescuers who go to the accident site must be fully equipped; standard equipment includes an avalanche transceiver worn on the body, probe and shovel, if possible also an avalanche airbag to avoid a complete burial or a breathing device (e.g. AvaLung) to be rescued in the event of a second-avalanche. It is quite legitimate to include the expected duration of a complete burial in the risk assessment and to assess the chances of survival depending on the time between the avalanche (or alarm) and the rescue and to weigh up the risk against the risk to the rescue teams. A short burial time (up to about 35 min) justifies a higher risk, after that the risk must be very carefully weighed up.

References

1. Falk M, Brugger H, Adler-Kastner L (1994) Avalanche survival chances. Nature 368:21
2. Soar J, Perkins GD, Abbas G, Alfonzo A, Barelli A, Bierens JJ, Brugger H, Deakin CD, Dunning J, Georgiou M, Handley AJ, Lockey DJ, Paal P, Sandroni C, Thies KC, Zideman DA, Nolan JP (2010) European Resuscitation Council guidelines for resuscitation 2010 section 8. Cardiac arrest in special circumstances: electrolyte abnormalities, poisoning, drowning, accidental hypothermia, hyperthermia, asthma, anaphylaxis, cardiac surgery, trauma, pregnancy, electrocution. Resuscitation 81:1400–1433
3. Brugger H, Durrer B, Adler-Kastner L, Falk M, Tschirky F (2001) Field management of avalanche victims. Resuscitation 51:7–15

ACS in 75-Year-old Patient

40

Peer G. Knacke

> ▶ Sometimes it is only a small hint, so to speak the "fine print", which provides the EMS team with a completely new differential diagnosis—as in this case, in which everything is literally not as it should normally be.

I have carried out over 15,000 missions as an emergency physician. At the first intervention today, the digital radio receiver shows next to the loud, hardly stoppable beeping on the display the keyword "ACS", i.e. an acute coronary syndrome. A classic that I have to take care of and that is not far away from the EMS station, so routine and certainly not terribly exciting. A few minutes after the alarm, we reach the emergency site, a beautifully located, very well-kept senior's residence with the option of additional care. Our patient is a 75-year-old, not seriously ill-looking, awake woman who takes care of herself and receives daily visits from the nursing service, which is also on site at the moment. When asked why an emergency physician was called, the patient reports about a dull pressure in the retrosternal area since the weekend. The question of radiation of the pain is answered with "in the left arm and in the legs". Then the nursing staff intervenes and says that the leg pain always exists, only the pain in the chest is new. The pain scale between 0 and 10 is answered with 2. The patient also has occasional chest pain, but also wetted herself last night, which does not usually happen. This actually sounds very confused! Auscultation of the lungs is uneventful, the heart sounds very quiet, the legs show slight edema on both sides. While trying to narrow down the acute symptomatology, the vital parameters are recorded in parallel. With the exception of hypertensive blood pressure values, these are uneventful (blood

P. G. Knacke (✉)
Department of Anesthesiology and Emergency Medicine, AMEOS Hospitals Ostholstein, Eutin, Germany
e-mail: p.knacke@t-online.de

V. Wenzel (ed.), *Case Studies in Emergency Medicine*,
https://doi.org/10.1007/978-3-662-67249-5_40

pressure 180/90 mmHg, heart rate 87/min, blood sugar 194 mg/dl, respiratory rate 14/min, oxygen saturation 100%), in addition, a 12-channel ECG is primary derived. This does not show any conspicuous repolarization disorders at a normofrequent absolute arrhythmia.

The nurse shows me a long list of prescriptions. It is originally sorted alphabetically, but here it is already sorted by drug groups for better overview: cardiovascular drugs (amlodipine, dihydralazine, metoprolol, glycerol trinitrate, digitoxin), diuretics (xipamide, torasemide, spironolactone), analgesics (morphine, novaminsulfone, oxycodone), the antiepileptic drug lamotrigine, the proton pump inhibitor pantoprazole, the bronchodilator tiotropium bromide, the anticoagulant rivaroxaban, and the psychopharmacon lorazepam. A truly proud list of medications, which also makes me think of drug interactions, since 25,000 people die from them in Germany every year (according to a report by the Süddeutsche Zeitung from 17.05.2010). But another drug shows me a clue: The patient takes the antiepileptic drug lamotrigine, has wetted the bed at night, and is otherwise not incontinent. Are the diuretics a problem or was it a seizure? The targeted inquiry reveals that the patient has been suffering from epilepsy since a stroke a few years ago. The last seizure was more than a year ago, so the regular intake of lamotrigine is taking place. A look at the tongue shows a classic lateral tongue bite. So at least we have a diagnosis: post-seizure enuresis at night. The current neurological finding is unspectacular. But is this compatible with the thoracic pressure? While I am just thinking about this question, the pager beeps again with the question of our possible availability for a heart attack in a neighboring town. The next physician-manned ambulance will need more than 20 min and the EMS helicopter is also not available. Since the patient we are currently treating is stable and her apartment is located near the hospital, this is confirmed with the stipulation that we can only start in about 4 min to finish therapy and documentation. After the already existing peripheral venous access, the patient receives two doses of nitroglycerin spray due to the complaints and the hypertensive circulatory situation.

While filling out the emergency medical services protocol and reviewing the patient file of the nursing service, I notice the small note "situs inversus". The patient is asked whether the organs are really arranged the wrong way around; she confirms this. The percussion confirms the dextrocardia—then we have to write the ECG mirror image. This surprises the present rescue assistants. In the ECG, there are clear ST depressions over the front wall as signs of ischemia. The patient now receives 5000 IE heparin and 250 mg aspirin intravenously, but she does not want an analgesic for the minor complaints. After being handed over to the ambulance, the patient is transported without problems to the nearby hospital, while we are on our way to the new assignment. The physician on duty of the local emergency room is informed by telephone about the assigned patient with the specialties.

Discussion

A situs inversus is a rare, non-pathological anatomical variant, which can however, as the case presented here shows, have consequences for diagnosis and therapy. In the first ECG, our patient showed a heart rhythm disorder, but no conduction disorders: These only became apparent in the adapted mirror image ECG. In the event of necessary defibrillation or transcutaneous pacemaker application, the electrodes would also have to be applied in a mirror image [1]. Even appendicitis would cause atypical symptoms in the left lower abdomen in the case of situs inversus. In the case of dextrocardia, the ECG does not show the typical increase in R-amplitude from V1–V6 in the normally glued chest lead, but the size of the QRS complexes becomes smaller to the left. A high R-amplitude in V1 is considered to be indicative of the diagnosis. If the two arm electrodes are swapped and V2–V1 and Vr3–Vr6 are derived instead of V1–V6, a normal ECG results for patients with situs inversus.

The diagnosis of a heart attack from the standard ECG and especially estimation of the infarct size and stages is often difficult in patients with unknown situs inversus [2].

40.1   Conclusion

In emergency diagnosis, it is easy to be wrong if you believe the first indications too much and are not alert when a finding does not fit the suspected diagnosis. It is important to form a consistent picture from the often complex picture of physical examination, medical history and the available written documents and to make a good diagnosis.

References

1. Shenthar J, Rai MK, Walia R, Ghanta S, Sreekumar P, Reddy SS (2014) Transvenous permanent pacemaker implantation in dextrocardia: technique, challenges, outcome, and a brief review of literature. Europace 16:1327–1333
2. Richter S, Doring M, Desch S, Hindricks G (2014) ECG pitfall: anterior myocardial infarction in dextrocardia. Eur Heart J 35:1887

Carried Off the Road

41

Hermann Brugger

▶ What to do if an emergency treatment has to be carried out, but one is not quite sure yet? And one does not know whether it really offers an optimal treatment condition for the intended transport? The present case provides answers to these questions.

At midnight the phone rings at the EMS operations center: operation in the Gader valley, traffic accident with several victims, injuries of unknown degree. In a few minutes we are on our way with the physician-manned ambulance with lights and sirens. The winding road into the Gader valley was built during the First World War, has seen many serious accidents and has been out of service for some time. At the time of the accident, a completely new route with numerous bridges and tunnels was built, the traffic was therefore redirected in one-way regulations via so-called "panoramic roads" on both sides of the valley over remote mountain villages and farms, which means a much longer journey time. After 45 min we reach the accident site at 1:00 a.m., at the end of a long curve. In front of a building there are already numerous emergency vehicles from the fire brigade, police and EMS. A large glass veranda of a restaurant is completely destroyed. In the middle of the guest room is a smashed sports car between tables, chairs and shards of glass. Firefighters are working on the car and removing the roof. One of the two people in the car has already been freed and is on the way to the hospital with minor injuries, the second is being lifted out of the car with the scoop stretcher as we arrive. I notice that the young man is unconscious but breathing and immediately have him brought to the physician-manned ambulance for treatment.

H. Brugger (✉)
EURAC Research, Institute of Mountain Emergency Medicine, Bozen, Italy
e-mail: hermann.brugger@eurac.edu

V. Wenzel (ed.), *Case Studies in Emergency Medicine*,
https://doi.org/10.1007/978-3-662-67249-5_41

The first examination reveals a Glasgow Coma Scale of 6 (1/1/4) with spontaneous respiration, oxygen saturation 88%, blood pressure 90/55 mmHg, sinus rhythm 95/min, unilateral dilated pupil right and an open fracture of the right thigh. Together with the paramedic, I insert a peripheral venous access, sedate and intubate the patient, check ventilation of both lungs and fix the tube. After the ventilator is turned on, I am just about to give the driver the go-ahead when the paramedic draws my attention to the oxygen saturation: 85%. After a few more minutes, oxygen saturation continues to drop to 78%, whereupon I temporarily stop departure to the hospital. I auscultate the lungs for the second time and can now no longer detect any respiratory sounds on the right. I vent the cuff and pull the endotracheal tube back slightly, assuming that I have mistakenly intubated the left main bronchus. On the other hand, this is actually unusual, I think to myself, because with a too low tube position, the tube normally comes to lie in the right bronchus trunk because it slopes more steeply. However, this new positioning does not change anything; I can still not auscultate any respiratory sounds over the right lung and the oxygen saturation is now only 72%. My working hypothesis is now that the patient has developed a tension pneumothorax on the right side and that circulation will fail parallel to the drop in oxygen saturation. I wonder if my surgical skills are sufficient for an emergency thoracic drainage. When working out the guidelines for the International Commission for Alpine Emergency Medicine ICAR MEDCOM [1], I learned the surgical approach. I am also aware of its indications in tension pneumothorax and multiple trauma patients, but so far this intervention has not been necessary in any of my missions. I fear that the patient will become cardiorespiratory unstable or even die during the expected long journey of about 45 min if we do not relieve the tension pneumothorax before we reach the hospital. My paramedic looks at me questioningly, I nod affirmatively and he already opens the surgical set and begins the preparations. After disinfection, I make a skin incision in the middle axillary line at the level of the right nipple, blunt the subcutaneous tissue with scissors, open the pleural space and, with the help of a finger, insert the thoracostomy tube with 28 Charrière into the pleural space. We attach a bladder catheter with urine bag to the tube, which immediately fills with air and some blood so that it has to be relieved with a cut. I fix the drainage provisionally with a stitch. After the saturation had fallen to 68% during the drainage and the blood pressure had fallen to 75/40 mmHg, both values now rise slowly and the saturation reaches an impressive 94% after about 10 min. The paramedic and I are relieved. We still connect the capnometer, which indicates end-expiratory carbon dioxide values of 35 mmHg, and set off. During the long journey, we monitor the patient, but he does not cause us any problems and we reach the hospital after three-quarters of an hour.

Discussion

The severe thoracic trauma is responsible for up to 25% of all fatal trauma [2]: an important form of therapy of the "Deadly Dozen" of a thoracic trauma is the relief of a tension pneumothorax with drainage. The pre-hospital emergency treatment of a tension pneumothorax is repeatedly discussed controversially in the literature [3]. In essence, two methods are available: needle puncture with catheter (>14 Charrière) in the second intercostal space in the mammillary line and surgical drainage with a thoracic drainage tube (28–36 Charrière) in the middle axillary line at the level of the nipple according to Bülau. Some authors are of the opinion that in an intubated patient with tension pneumothorax and cardiorespiratory insufficiency, surgical relief by means of a large drainage for venting the needle puncture is superior [4]. The use of a sharp trocar in emergency medicine should be avoided because of the risk of injury to thoracic organs [3]. A valve supply (Heimlich valve) is not necessary during mechanical ventilation. Some basic thoughts: if a simple pneumothorax is found in a non-intubated emergency patient, this does not necessarily mean the need for action. If the oxygen saturation is acceptable, the circulation is stable and the patient is not intubation-dependent, pre-hospital relief of the pneumothorax is not necessary. If, on the other hand, a patient with a simple pneumothorax is intubated and ventilated, the probability is very high that a tension pneumothorax will develop with the risk of cardiorespiratory instability due to displacement of the mediastinum to the healthy side. This can happen very quickly and then the situation becomes acutely dangerous. In these cases, it may be that puncture with small-caliber catheters in a reasonable time no longer has the desired effect, especially if it is a multiple trauma patient who has to be brought to a trauma center for surgical repair as quickly as possible. Delayed action or half-hearted steps should be avoided, that is, in this case it is advisable to seek efficient and lasting relief quickly. It should also be kept in mind that auscultation of the lungs is hardly possible due to the noise level on the way, especially if you are in a helicopter. During a helicopter transport, it should also be kept in mind in advance that during the ascent, for example when flying over passes or ridges, the circulatory situation can deteriorate during the flight due to the intrapleural relative increase in pressure, precisely when no therapy is possible during the flight [5]. It is therefore better to carry out both the diagnosis and the therapy of a pneumothorax before flying to the hospital.

In order not to endanger the patient when setting up a thoracic drainage, the personal experience of the emergency physician must always be taken into account; there are fatal complications of thoracic drainage in the literature, for example by laceration of large vessels, the heart, the lung or the liver [6]. In an analysis of emergency calls in Baden-Württemberg/Germany, EMS helicopter physicians inserted a thoracic drainage every 6 months, but emergency physicians in ground-based EMS vehicles only every 77 months (approximately 6.5 years) [7]. This rare use of a potentially dangerous, but also life-saving intervention such as thoracic drainage shows that the emergency physician should make a good assessment of the patient's clinical condition, his own manual skills and experience as well as the availability of more experienced colleagues—whether in another EMS vehicle or in the next hospital.

One year after the accident, I receive a call in my practice: "Chiamo da Milano e sono il padre del ragazzo …" It is the father of the injured person who informs us that his 18-year-old son had to be neurologically rehabilitated for months, but can now lead a normal life again and passed the final exams the day before. Not only to his, but also to my great joy.

41.1 Conclusion

For the treatment of trauma patients, one should always be trained and prepared for the relief of a tension pneumothorax, and above all take a tension pneumothorax into a differential diagnosis. You can expect this especially after endotracheal intubation with mechanical ventilation. The lateral surgical approach is particularly advantageous over the relief with needles if respiration or circulation is severely impaired, high altitudes are reached or a long transport is pending.

References

1. Forster H, Zafren K (2007) Thoracostomy at the scene of an accident in the mountains. ICAR MEDCOM recommendation 12. http://www.ikar-cisa.org/ikar-cisa/documents/2007/RECM0012E.pdf. Accessed: 5. Mar 2015
2. Cipolle M, Rhodes M, Tinkoff G (2012) Deadly dozen: dealing with the 12 types of thoracic injuries. JEMS 37:60–65
3. Barton ED, Epperson M, Hoyt DB, Fortlage D, Rosen P (1995) Prehospital needle aspiration and tube thoracostomy in trauma victims: a six-year experience with aeromedical crews. J Emerg Med 13:155–163
4. Martin M, Satterly S, Inaba K, Blair K (2012) Does needle thoracostomy provide adequate and effective decompression of tension pneumothorax? J Trauma Acute Care Surg 73:1412–1417
5. Braude D, Tutera D, Tawil I, Pirkl G (2014) Air transport of patients with pneumothorax: is tube thoracostomy required before flight? Air Med J 33:152–156
6. Schley M, Rossler M, Konrad CJ, Schupfer G (2009) Damage of the subclavian vein with a thorax drainage. Anaesthesist 58:387–390
7. Gries A, Zink W, Bernhard M, Messelken M, Schlechtriemen T (2006) Realistic assessment of the physician-staffed emergency services in Germany. Anaesthesist 55:1080–1086

Dangerous EMS Scene Call

42

Volker Wenzel

▶ Physicians are in an enormous responsibility and not always make or transmit the patients and their relatives decisions or results, which they would like to hear. And that can—quite not rarely—lead to situations that can be life-threatening for the physicians themselves.

The physician-manned ambulance is alarmed early Saturday morning to a pub on the outskirts of the city with the message "unconscious person". A typical mission at this time and on this day of the week, only the locations change during the night towards the bars, which offer breakfast as well. Depending on the size of the area, each doctor has such a scene call on weekends, insofar as the emergency physician expects nothing special on the way to this emergency. Arrived at the scene, a man of about 30 years is already in the ambulance next to a café, which is very popular with motorcycle clubs. According to information from the paramedics, the vital parameters are stable. Witnesses report that the drunk patient was involved in a fight and after a blow to the chest fell backwards, hit his head on the street and then became unconscious. Since the patient does not react to address, nor to touch, the emergency physician begins with the body check, whereby she finds injuries in the face. When trying to open the eyes for an examination of the pupils, the patient suddenly begins to fight. The emergency physician steps back, but too late—she is hit by the patient's fist with full force in the neck area. Neither the emergency physician herself nor the present paramedics can react so quickly to prevent the fist. The restless patient is taken to the local hospital for treatment

V. Wenzel (✉)
Department of Anesthesiology, Intensive Care, Emergency Medicine and Pain Therapy, Friedrichshafen Regional Medical Center and Tettnang Hospital, Friedrichshafen / Tettnang, Germany
e-mail: v.wenzel@klinikum-fn.de

V. Wenzel (ed.), *Case Studies in Emergency Medicine*,
https://doi.org/10.1007/978-3-662-67249-5_42

of alcohol intoxication and facial injuries. The emergency physician herself ends her shift several hours later with mild headaches and neck pain. Only after several days later, visual impairments occur and the headaches become stronger, the emergency physician also goes to the hospital for neurological examination. A dissection of the carotid artery with functional closure on the side struck by the fist and a dissection of the vertebral artery on the contralateral side is diagnosed. The emergency physician is immediately admitted to the stroke unit and heparinized to prevent a stroke. Afterwards she is six weeks unable to work. For months she is anticoagulated and the neck vessels are continuously controlled. In the end, the dissection regresses and the emergency physician can continue her work in anesthesia. However, there is one thing she will probably never do again in her life—work as an emergency physician in a physician-manned ambulance.

The perpetrator of the injury remains unpunished from a criminal point of view, as at the time of the punch he could not assess the consequences of his action due to alcohol intoxication and a concussion. He is acquitted at the trial. What remains is very annoyed paramedics and EMS physicians.

Discussion

Aggressions against physicians have been described when healthcare has not kept pace with population growth and thus ever-increasing numbers of patients are coming into contact with ever-more overworked physicians [1]. In January 2015, a man went to Brigham's and Women's Hospital in Boston, USA, to speak to the cardiac surgeon who had operated on his mother. When the cardiac surgeon entered the consultation room, the patient's son pulled out a gun and immediately shot the cardiac surgeon twice and then shot himself. Despite emergency surgery, the cardiac surgeon, a father of three children, could not be saved. Suddenly, American physicians became aware of how vulnerable they are to possible aggressions by patients disappointed with their treatment in a country with more than 300 million firearms in private hands [2]. In a study in the USA, there were a total of 154 shootings in hospitals (91) or on hospital premises (63) between 2000 and 2011, resulting in the deaths of 24 hospital staff, 12 nurses, 8 doctors and 4 pharmacists [3]. In autumn 2013, the police in Lower Austria were on the trail of a poacher; at a police roadblock, the poacher immediately opened fire on the officers, seriously injuring a policeman, and then fled into the forest. About 1 h later, he shot a paramedic who was driving an ambulance to take the seriously injured policeman to hospital. Another hour later, the poacher stopped a police patrol car and shot the two policemen; later, he shot himself in his house (*Kurier* 18.09.2013).

In a survey of doctors working in emergency departments in Michigan, USA, 75% of doctors said they had been verbally attacked in the last 12 months; 28% said they had already been physically attacked, 12% had been confronted by patients outside the emergency department and 4% had been stalked by patients. Accordingly, 82% of these doctors said they sometimes feel afraid of violence at work [4]. If one believes that violence against doctors only occurs in overloaded healthcare systems or in societies with extremely high levels of privately owned firearms, one is wrong—doctors and paramedics are regularly and increasingly being physically attacked in German-speaking countries, with emergency departments, out-of-hours medical services, emergency medical services and work in social hotspots being the most dangerous. As shocked as those involved in aggressions against physicians are, so little is said about it; possibly because of heightened and misguided professional ideals that "a good and empathetic doctor is not attacked" (*Northern Lights current* 09/2014). This is simply not true because even in German-speaking countries (with extremely strict laws for guns in private hands) physicians become victims of serious violence, many of them with fatal outcome [5]. A neurologist and psychiatrist in Saarbrücken, Germany was shot by one of her patients in her own office (*Frankfurter Allgemeine Zeitung* 13.03.2015), an EMS helicopter in Upper Austria was blinded by a laser upon landing on the hospital roof (*Die Presse* 18.08.2011), a drunk man in Berlin, Germany stabbed a knife into the neck of a helping paramedic (*Tagesspiegel* 06.08.2007), an ambulance driver from Freising, Germany got a punch in the face from the friend of an emergency patient in Fürstenfeldbruck, Germany, and passers-by shot fireworks at firefighters who wanted to extinguish a fire (*Süddeutsche Zeitung* 10.01.2012). These cases should only be the tip of an iceberg of violence against people in the healthcare industry, if one reads the accounts of hospital employees in southern Germany (*Süddeutsche Zeitung* 09.02.2015). In the Center for Sleep Medicine in Nuremberg, a senior physician was beaten several times in the face because the cure demanded by a patient was refused by a psychosomatic hospital. In the emergency room of the Ingolstadt Hospital, two rival groups went at each other; eight nurses had to be called to resolve the situation. "In the end, everything was full of blood," said a witness. A hospital spokeswoman said: "In psychiatric hospitals, there has always been such an aggression potential, but now even hospitals of basic care are not spared." In emergency rooms, it is now "attention to remove everything that can be misused as a projectile." A physician in a Nuremberg Hospital in Germany says, "that the progressing barbarism of society does not stop at the hospital—our physicians were long protected by the white coat—but that is over." In the same hospital, a resident physician had to flee in front of 20 relatives in the geriatrics ward, but could lock herself in a patient's room. As the author of the Süddeutsche Zeitung wrote on 09.02.2015, in German hospitals "barking, threatening, beating and fondling" is present; but exact numbers are difficult to obtain. It is only certain that aggressions arise more from male and intoxicated patients. With age, one can not predict anything anymore, because even 80-year-olds suddenly strike, as an analysis showed. In a study by the Ruhr-University in Bochum, Germany, 900 paramedics and firefighters were interviewed; almost everyone was already exposed to verbal attacks, 59% also to aggressive attacks and 25% also to criminal violence—in the last twelve months. While hospitals are happy to communicate any new technology in detail, security aspects are rather adapted silently—employees are sent to deescalation training or nurses train in self-defense courses how they can escape from chokeholds patient-friendly and security guards are mainly used at night to contain aggressions.

42.1 Conclusion

Verbal and physical violence against physicians has increased and is more common in the treatment of intoxicated or psychotic patients than in the treatment of "normal" patients. But even over the course of treatment or with treatment considered disadvantageous, frustrated patients or their relatives can suddenly attack physicians, EMS and hospital staff, the health consequences of which can be severe. In an emergency scene call, look for opportunities or safe rooms to protect yourself from a sudden attack by the patient, relatives or bystanders. Individual protection can be improved by a self-defense course; a zero risk is not possible with open hospital doors and emergency physicians responding to emergency locations without security screening. Physicians should demand prevention measures against violence from their hospital, emergency medical and EMS providers.

References

1. Xu W (2014) Violence against doctors in China. Lancet 384:745
2. Rosenbaum L (2015) Being like Mike-fear, trust, and the tragic death of Michael Davidson. N Engl J Med 372:798–799
3. Kelen GD, Catlett CL, Kubit JG, Hsieh YH (2012) Hospital-based shootings in the United States: 2000 to 2011. Ann Emerg Med 60:790–798, e791
4. Kowalenko T, Walters BL, Khare RK, Compton S (2005) Workplace violence: a survey of emergency physicians in the state of Michigan. Ann Emerg Med 46:142–147
5. Maulen B (2013) An ever increasing incidence of violence against physicians. MMW Fortschr Med 155:14–16, 18, 20

Shortness of Breath in Steam Room 43

Norman Hecker and Bernd Domres

▶ Not everything is as it seems and what it seems—as this case very clearly shows. That is why a sound differential diagnosis is very important, as well as the saying, "when you hear hooves, think horses … and maybe zebras."

There are often reports of deployment that suggest the suspicion of an acute coronary syndrome on the way to the deployment site. One of the most common deployment reports in the emergency medical service are "chest pain and shortness of breath", often with an acute coronary syndrome. The term acute coronary syndrome includes the classic myocardial infarction (STEMI; ST-segment elevation myocardial infarction), the non-ST-segment elevation myocardial infarction (NSTEMI; non-ST-segment elevation myocardial infarction) and unstable angina pectoris. While the STEMI can be diagnosed relatively safely and clearly in the pre-hospital phase and treated accordingly in accordance with the applicable guidelines, the pre-hospital diagnosis of the other two disease patterns is much more difficult and therefore much more dependent on the experience of the emergency physician. All 3 disease patterns are the same in principle. Typically, these are devastating pains in the chest area, shortness of breath and heart rhythm disorders, cold sweats, dizziness, nausea, vomiting or even a circulatory collapse are unspecific, but often associated symptoms. Depending on other pre-existing conditions, milder and less clear courses and causes can occur with the typical

N. Hecker (✉)
Department of Emergency Medicine, Protestant Hospital, Gelsenkirchen, Germany
e-mail: hecker@evk-ge.de

B. Domres
Foundation of the German Institute for Disaster Medicine, Tübingen, Germany
e-mail: bddomres@yahoo.de

© The Author(s), under exclusive license to Springer-Verlag GmbH, DE, part of Springer Nature 2023
V. Wenzel (ed.), *Case Studies in Emergency Medicine*,
https://doi.org/10.1007/978-3-662-67249-5_43

symptoms; so it can be anything between psychosomatic complaints and a fatal myocardial infarction.

On a cold winter day, the emergency dispatch center receives a call for help from the local hot spring. The caller, an employee of the facility, reports that a woman in her middle years has collapsed in the steam room and is groaning in pain, gasping for air. As a result, the emergency physician-manned ambulance and an ambulance manned by two paramedics are alerted. Upon arrival, the EMS team encounters a 53-year-old, approximately 165 cm tall, obese woman who is responsive but not fully oriented and dazed. She has cold, sweaty skin, shortness of breath, and reports a pressing pain in the epigastrium that radiates to the chest, back, and left arm, which has been getting worse since this morning after breakfast. The patient fell due to dizziness, but never lost consciousness. There are no known pre-existing conditions, although blood pressure may have been "high at times" in the past and she smokes about 15 cigarettes, often when drinking coffee. Blood pressure is 110/60 mmHg, ECG shows a sinus rhythm with a rate of 58/min with no ST-segment elevation, there are occasional supraventricular extrasystoles, peripheral oxygen saturation is 98% with 17–20 breaths per minute. There are no contusions on the thorax, the abdomen is distended and mildly tender to palpation in all 4 quadrants without guarding, both kidney areas are free of percussion pain, the rest of the body check is negative. After taking the history and physical examination, the working diagnosis of "acute coronary syndrome—suspicion of NSTEMI" is made by the emergency physician. Differential diagnoses include a collapse due to syncope (e.g. due to cardiac forward failure with sudden peripheral vasodilation from the hot thermal water) or a dissection of a large vessel. The emergency physician initiates symptomatic therapy with volume, antiemetics, oxygen, an analgesic, and monitoring. The patient is then transported with the emergency physician-manned ambulance accompanying the patient onboard to the nearest hospital that has surgery, but no invasive cardiology.

There are good reasons to follow the working diagnosis of the emergency physician in this case. On the one hand, the patient reports the classical leading symptom of a myocardial infarction; namely, thoracic pain radiating to adjacent regions. Pain radiation to the arms or shoulders is typical of a myocardial infarction [1] and helps to distinguish it from other causes [2]. Other symptoms such as shortness of breath and cold sweats are also characteristic. In particular, if these symptoms are combined with atypical symptoms such as nausea and collapse in women, the suspicion of an acute myocardial infarction is likely [3]. On the other hand, there is no ST elevation, but an extrasystole. Various ECG changes can indicate or simulate a myocardial infarction, even in the absence of ST elevation [4, 5]. In combination with the clinical examination findings, the working diagnosis of "acute coronary syndrome—suspicion of NSTEMI" appears justified. The clinical examination confirms the findings of the emergency physician, in particular the epigastric pain radiating to the thoracic region and the intermittent extrasystole in the ECG; the admitting internist therefore takes over the working diagnosis of the emergency physician. However, the laboratory-chemical examination shows a normal blood analysis, creatine kinase 122 U/L, CK-MB 7 U/L and troponin-T

0.12 µg/L. This laboratory-chemical analysis combined with the lack of elevations in the EKG excludes an acute myocardial infarction as the cause of the symptoms with sufficient high certainty.

The actual decision of the emergency physician and the admitting internist to diagnose a myocardial infarction is basically understandable and comprehensible. A newly occurring angina pectoris is considered unstable angina pectoris and would therefore remain open as a possible differential diagnosis. In our case, however, it is not an acute coronary syndrome, but the effect of a massive stomach distension—shortly after the patient was admitted to the hospital, she had to vomit several times. This is because she had drunk large amounts of latte macchiato shortly before visiting the spa with a friend. Since she has been suffering from constipation for years, this results in the diagnosis of a Roemheld syndrome [6]. The patient recovers quickly after symptomatic therapy.

Discussion
In the Roemheld syndrome, the diaphragm is raised directly or indirectly due to a passage disorder or bloating in the gastrointestinal tract and thus exerts mechanical pressure on the heart [6]. The symptomatology of the Roemheld syndrome can thus simulate the clinical picture of angina pectoris in a surprising way; fortunately, in contrast to the "real" acute coronary syndrome, the cause is often harmless and easy to fix. For the emergency doctor, it is essential that myocardial infarctions are time-critical events whose extent of damage and prognosis benefit significantly from early and guideline-based therapy initiation. Even if not every suspicion of an acute coronary syndrome is a real acute coronary syndrome, the rapid clarification of a suspicion of NSTEMI or unstable angina pectoris seems urgently necessary. The Roemheld syndrome is certainly not the typical differential diagnosis for acute coronary syndrome, but our case shows that despite the clinical and economic importance of acute coronary syndrome, one must always think of other possible causes. While we instill the motto in our medical students that one should "think of horses and not zebras when one hears hoofbeats" [7], this helps to separate the probable from the improbable, but of course it cannot replace the expertise of the emergency doctor to make decisions in complex situations. In a case with thoracic pain, a heart rate of 170/min, consciousness disturbance and ST-segment elevation, the patient was treated with the suspicion of a STEMI with aspirin, heparin and clopidogrel and brought to the cardiac catheterization laboratory, where no pathology of the coronary arteries was found, but the diagnosis of a Brugada syndrome. The authors concluded that when you hear hoofbeats, you should think of horses **and** zebras [8]. In a Dutch study of 820 patients with the suspicion of a STEMI who were referred to a university hospital for cardiology for percutaneous invasive intervention, 19 patients (2.3%) ultimately had no STEMI, but pericarditis (5), aortic dissection (3), subarachnoid hemorrhage (2), cardiomyopathy (2), pneumonia (1), COPD (1), mediastinal tumor (1),

peritonitis (1), Brugada syndrome (1), coronary aneurysm (1) or aortic stenosis (1). Tragically, the patients with aortic dissection and subarachnoid hemorrhage were also anticoagulated because of the suspicion of a STEMI and died [9].

43.1 Conclusion

The difficulty for the prehospital emergency physician is to ensure the rapid start of therapy in the event of a manifest suspicion of an acute coronary syndrome (so-called "Golden Hour"), but at the same time to choose the clinical place of treatment so that differential diagnoses can also be treated. Therefore, non-cardiac causes, and thus, for example, surgical diseases, must also be considered. Here we remember aortic dissection, hiatal hernia and pneumothorax. However, in the event of a high suspicion of an acute heart attack, coronary intervention remains the essential therapeutic element.

References

1. Albarran J, Durham B, Gowers J, Dwight J, Chappell G (2002) Is the radiation of chest pain a useful indicator of myocardial infarction? A prospective study of 541 patients. Accid Emerg Nurs 10:2–9
2. Sanchis J, Bodi V, Nunez J, Bosch X, Heras M, Bonanad C, Pellicer M, Merlos P, Minana G, Llacer A (2011) Usefulness of pain presentation characteristics for predicting outcome in patients presenting to the hospital with chest pain of uncertain origin. Emerg Med J 28:847–850
3. Coventry LL, Finn J, Bremner AP (2011) Sex differences in symptom presentation in acute myocardial infarction: a systematic review and meta-analysis. Heart Lung 40:477–491
4. Wang K, Asinger RW, Marriott HJ (2003) ST-segment elevation in conditions other than acute myocardial infarction. N Engl J Med 349:2128–2135
5. Yahalom M, Roguin N, Suleiman K, Turgeman Y (2013) Clinical significance of conditions presenting with ECG changes mimicking acute myocardial infarction. Int J Angiol 22:115–122
6. Janner J (1956) Aerophagia and abdominal distention; Roemheld, Chilaiditi splenic flexure syndrome. Schweiz Med Wochenschr 86:886–891
7. Beales D (2008) Hoofbeats. Ann Intern Med 148:164–165
8. Hudzik B, Szkodzinski J, Wozniak A, Nowowiejska-Wiewiora A, Polonski L (2011) When you hear hoofbeats, think of horses and zebras: a 58-year-old man with chest pain and palpitations. Intern Emerg Med 6:537–541
9. Gu YL, Svilaas T, van der Horst IC, Zijlstra F (2008) Conditions mimicking acute ST-segment elevation myocardial infarction in patients referred for primary percutaneous coronary intervention. Neth Heart J 16:325–331

Swallow and Brake Failure

44

Hermann Brugger

▶ When is a CPR really useful? And when should it be waited for? In addition to this question, the present case puts the focus on how important it is to secure the patient as well as the self-protection in the EMS.

I am currently checking the expiration dates of the drugs in the emergency medical kits with an ambulance driver and notice in the background that the EMS vehicle is being dispatched. Minutes later, the alarm sounds. "Circulatory arrest in a small mountain village". This settlement is a remote mountain village (elevation, 1.500 m / 4,900 feet above sea level) with a dozen farms, reachable in the best case in 20 min by a steep, winding road from our EMS station. The area made headlines in the 1960s when, in a wild raid, all male residents were taken away by police and military and numerous houses were set on fire because a village was suspected of being involved in bomb attacks against the Italian "occupation" of South Tyrol. For a long time this area has been suffering from emigration, but also from depressions and substance abuse. I had been called as a general practitioner to certify the death of a single farmer who had hanged himself in his living room only shortly before.

Since our regular regular physician-manned ambulance is in repair, we have to go out today with a replacement physician-manned ambulance. The van is spacious, but it has already been on the road for many years and has racked up a lot of mileage, and it winds its way up the steep road to the scene of the accident at a maximum speed of 40–50 km/h (25–31 mph). I estimate that we will need about 20 min to get there, and that the chances of saving the patient are tending towards zero. When we reach the farm and enter the living room, I see a man in his early

H. Brugger (✉)
EURAC Research, Institute for Mountain Emergency Medicine, Bozen, Italy
e-mail: hermann.brugger@eurac.edu

191

V. Wenzel (ed.), *Case Studies in Emergency Medicine*,
https://doi.org/10.1007/978-3-662-67249-5_44

fifties lying on the floor and the EMS team performing cardiopulmonary resuscitation. There are no relatives to be seen. I am told that the patient was already motionless when the first team arrived, so an unobserved circulatory arrest, and, as expected, probably very poor prospects.

I immediately order preparation for endotracheal intubation. I am greatly surprised when, during laryngoscopy, I see that the glottis is closed by a finger-thick piece of meat. With the Magill forceps, I pull the foreign body out like a champagne cork, insert the tube into the trachea and ventilate with 100% oxygen. The ECG shows asystole. It is worth trying with epinephrine and shortly thereafter, a sinus bradycardia sets in. After another 1 mg dose of adrenaline, the heart frequency normalizes, a carotid pulse can finally be palpated and a systolic blood pressure of 90 mmHg can be measured. We wait a few more minutes for the stabilization of circulation and then decide on a quick transport to the hospital.

After we brought the patient into the physician-manned ambulance, we set off downhill: The driver at the wheel, the paramedic in the cabin and me with the patient. There are no complications, the heart is beating rhythmically, the cardiac performance is sufficient, I am more than satisfied, when on one of the steepest sections of the road the car suddenly picks up speed, becomes faster and faster and the driver turns around and shouts "hey Doc, the brakes have failed!" I think now we have saved the patient and everyone falls into the abyss—instead of one dead, there are maybe 4 dead! We immediately set ourselves with our backs to the direction of travel against the wall of the cabin (the patient is anyway strapped in) and hope that the driver will still get the situation under control. And indeed, the professional truck driver and voluntary paramedic manages to reduce the speed by shifting and operating the handbrake so that he can cope with the steep section with the engine brake. However, now we only continue in first gear and a speed of 20 km/h (12.4 mph), so we need almost 40 min to reach the hospital. To top it all off, we also crash into a concrete pillar in the underground car park on the way into the hospital. We reach the emergency room quite exhausted from this horror ride and hand over the still circulatory stable patient.

Discussion

There are, against all statistics, sometimes exceptions to the rule. It is known that a normothermic patient cannot survive a circulatory arrest for more than 10–15 min. When estimating the chance of survival of a circulatory arrest, we often assume a cardiac cause, where this deadline actually applies. In this case, however, the circulatory arrest was not due to a cardiac cause, but to an asphyxia caused by a high-sitting bolus. An obstruction of the airways leads to alveolar hypoxia, coronary hypoperfusion and secondary to cardiac circulatory arrest. Experimental studies have shown that up to the onset of pulselessness 3 to 10 min can pass [1, 2] and the time from the event to asystole can take up to 20 min [3]. It is also not excluded that in our case the bolus did not hermetically seal the airway and thus extended this "gallows period".

The vehicles of the emergency medical service also take part in road traffic and can thus be involved in an accident, especially when driving with lights and sirens—regularly one reads reports about it in the newspaper. Again and again we observe that physicians and paramedics do not fasten their seat belts, especially when accompanying a patient in the physician-manned ambulance. It should be noted that there are many corners and edges in the patient compartment of a physician-manned ambulance, which can cause considerable injuries if, for example, one is thrown against it in an accident. The most important thing: While we show our students that they have to pay attention to their own protection at an accident site in addition to saving lives, we are often careless in everyday emergency medical care. In Tyrol / Austria, the driver of an ambulance was charged with negligent homicide because he drove into a car, causing the transported patient to be so seriously injured that she eventually died; (ORF, 11.04.2012) on the Internet you can quickly find similar cases.

44.1 Conclusion

If there is a suspicion of obstructive asphyxia when finding an unconscious person, one should also be careful in the assessment of the chances of success of cardiopulmonary resuscitation in the event of an unobserved cardiac arrest and not regard longer time intervals from circulatory collapse to the beginning of CPR as hopeless. This mainly affects bolus death, but also avalanche burial [3] and hanging. In general, this case confirms that an optimistic attitude is not wrong in these resuscitation situations. But it also shows that in emergency medicine one always has to expect everything, one is never safe from surprises and emergency physicians can sometimes be exposed to unpredictable risks. Sometimes it takes a good portion of luck to bring both the patient and oneself safely into port. One should never forget self-protection.

References

1. Safar P, Paradis NA, Weil MH (2007) Asphyxial cardiac arrest. In: Paradis NA, Halperin HR, Kern KB, Wenzel V, Chamberlain DA (Hrsg) Cardiac arrest – the science and practice of resuscitation medicine. Cambridge University Press, Cambridge, S 969–993
2. Varvarousi G, Xanthos T, Lappas T, Lekka N, Goulas S, Dontas I, Perrea D, Stefanadis C, Papadimitriou L (2011) Asphyxial cardiac arrest, resuscitation and neurological outcome in a Landrace/Large-white swine model. Lab Anim 45(3):184–190
3. Heschl S, Paal P, Farzi S (2013) Electrical cardiac activity in an avalanche victim dying of asphyxia. Resuscitation 84:e143–144

Injury From Power Line

45

Jan Breckwoldt

▶ There are topics that are underrepresented in emergency medical theory and practice, and communication of "bad news" definitely and unfortunately falls into that category. This case provides some helpful approaches to deal with it.

Late one beautiful summer day—not too hot, not too cold—we fly to a large forest with our EMS helicopter. In addition to the approximate location of the incident, our only information is "SI" (Severe Injury). From the air, we can see an ambulance near a single-track railway line in a pine and birch forest, with two paramedics and a person lying on the ground near it; other than that, there is nothing but forest as far as the eye can see. We land a short distance from the railway track and make our way up a gentle hill. Now we see a ladder against an overhead power line of the railway, from which the high-voltage technician has fallen about 5 m. As far as we can determine, the patient had contact with 14,000 V of electricity and then fell onto the relatively soft forest floor; a body check reveals no indications of fractures of the large bones.

The patient is awake and responding appropriately; when asked, he reports severe pain in his right leg but also in the corresponding arm. The right trouser leg and right boot are completely charred, the affected extremity is completely stiff, and the right hand shows clear signs of electrical burns. The patient cannot give any account of the accident, but the pattern of injuries suggests that the 14,000 V from the overhead power line completely traversed the right side of the patient's body, causing severe thermal damage to the internal organs in the process. I have treated some patients with such severe electrical injuries in the course of my years in the emergency room of our university hospital, and I have always

J. Breckwoldt (✉)
University Hospital, Department of Anesthesiology, Zürich, Switzerland
e-mail: jan.breckwoldt@usz.ch

V. Wenzel (ed.), *Case Studies in Emergency Medicine*,
https://doi.org/10.1007/978-3-662-67249-5_45

been very affected by how clear-headed these patients were shortly after the electrical accident, even though they had an injury that was almost certainly fatal. Mechanistically, it was clear what needed to be done for this patient in the forest: analgesia and air transport to the burn center. Because of the possible hallucinogenic side effects, not to mention the bright sunlight and the subsequent helicopter transport, I ruled out the option of ketamine for spontaneous respiration. So we prepared for general anesthesia. While I was talking to the patient, I had the feeling that he did not understand at all how serious his situation was I certainly wouldn't want to bet on it, but I was convinced of an absolutely bleak prognosis. Should I tell him? In the end, I decided against it, opting instead to get him pain-free and conscious for this beautiful summer day. We then titrated the patient with fentanyl until he was pain-free. When I asked him, just before induction of anesthesia, to imagine something very beautiful, he spoke of his wife and children. Then he fell asleep. For me, it was clear that these were probably the last thoughts in his life.

He later died of the consequences of his injuries in the burn center, without ever regaining consciousness.

The question that went through my head at the time, I still can't answer for sure. How "honest" should we be with the patients entrusted to us, especially when our contact is short and brief, as is so often the case in emergency medicine? In the end, I made the decision at the time because I thought it wouldn't have made any difference either way - neither for the patient nor for the relatives. But maybe he could have left an important message for his family? And was I really sure with my prognosis? And could I really have conveyed the situation to him in such a short time? If I were in such a situation again, I would probably ask if I should pass on a message to his wife.

> **Discussion**
> A Medline search for the question of what and how to communicate "bad news" in emergency medicine only provides results for communicating with relatives [1], while disciplines such as oncology, in which patients are accompanied for years, have a lot of experience with direct communication with the patient [2]. Why communication of "bad news" in emergency medicine is extremely difficult becomes clear when looking at the probably most widespread model for conveying bad news, the SIPKES model [3]. In this 6-step model, the conversation is first prepared spatially and in content ("Setting"), then it is asked what the patient and possibly his family already know ("[patient's] Perception"), it is checked how the information is to be handled ("Invitation") and only then it is announced that "bad news" are to be conveyed, including the specific content ("[provide] Knowledge"). In the following steps, the emotions are processed ("[addressing] Emotions") and the goals and priorities for further treatment and the exact plan of how this is to be achieved are set ("Strategy and Summary") [3]. Such a step-by-step and careful communication is not possible in emergency medicine, on the

one hand because of the blatant time pressure and on the other hand because an accurate prognosis often cannot be estimated. For the - certainly easier - communication with relatives in the field of emergency medicine, however, the SPIKES model offers a good basis and corresponding content has now been included in emergency medical training [4] and in student curricula [5]. Incidentally, a study on conveying "bad news" in the emergency room showed that the communication process was perceived more positively by the relatives than by the physicians who conveyed the news [6].

For direct communication with dying emergency patients, orientation to a stepwise model appears to be less suitable. Nevertheless, even in a short time window, we can send positive signals to patients and their relatives and avoid negative messages. As a patient cared for by hematooncologists in Boston wrote, "you should never say 'we can't do anything more for you,' this ignores, the treatment of pain and creates a feeling of being completely lost." [7] Two oncologists from Germany also consider communicating bad news to be one of the most difficult, but also one of the most important medical task, regardless of the specialty. In their article, they explain the decisive influence that communicative skills have on the subjective well-being of patients and their relatives, as well as on compliance, emotional disease processing and the ability to make decisions. [8].

The Swiss writer and architect Max Frisch wrote: "One should hold the truth out to the other like a coat for him to slip into, and not slap it around his ears like a wet rag." [9] How we can best proceed under the special conditions of emergency medicine in short conversations with patients and their relatives is answered by general practitioners from Houston, Texas: "Hope is always important for people. Physicians should convey hope without raising unrealistic expectations." [10]

45.1 Conclusion

Breaking bad news in emergency medicine is very difficult due to the time pressure, unclear prognosis and largely absent intimacy. Instead, positive communication should be used and hope should be conveyed, without raising unrealistic hopes. If a patient with fatal injuries is still conscious before induction of anesthesia, it is possible to ask whether any information should be passed to the relatives.

References

1. Limehouse WE, Feeser VR, Bookman KJ, Derse A (2012) A model for emergency department end-of-life communications after acute devastating events–part I: decision-making capacity, surrogates, and advance directives. Acad Emerg Med 19:E1068–E1072

2. Cherny NI (2011) Factors influencing the attitudes and behaviors of oncologists regarding the truthful disclosure of information to patients with advanced and incurable cancer. Psychooncology 20:1269–1284
3. Baile WF, Buckman R, Lenzi R, Glober G, Beale EA, Kudelka AP (2000) SPIKES – a six-step protocol for delivering bad news: application to the patient with cancer. Oncologist 5:302–311
4. Servotte JC, Bragard I, Szyld D, Van Ngoc P, Scholtes B, Van Cauwenberge I, Donneau AF, Dardenne N, Goosse M, Pilote B, Guillaume M, Ghuysen A (2019) Efficacy of a short role-play training on breaking bad news in the emergency department. West J Emerg Med 20:893–902
5. Bächli P, Meindl-Fridez C, Weiss-Breckwoldt AN, Breckwoldt J. (2019) Challenging cases during clinical clerkships beyond the domain of the „medical expert": an analysis of students' case vignettes. GMS J Med Educ 36:Doc30
6. Toutin-Dias G, Daglius-Dias R, Scalabrini-Neto A (2018) Breaking bad news in the emergency department: a comparative analysis among residents, patients and family members' perceptions. Eur J Emerg Med 25:71–76
7. Dias L, Chabner BA, Lynch TJ Jr, Penson RT (2003) Breaking bad news: a patient's perspective. Oncologist 8:587–596
8. Schilling G, Mehnert A (2014) Breaking bad news–a challenge for every physician. Med Klin Intensivmed Notfmed 109:609–613
9. Frisch M (1983) Die Tagebücher, 1946–1949. Suhrkamp, Berlin, S 1966–1971
10. Whitney SN, McCullough LB, Fruge E, McGuire AL, Volk RJ (2008) Beyond breaking bad news: the roles of hope and hopefulness. Cancer 113:442–445

Person Trapped

46

Frank Marx

▶ "Making decisions prospectively is much harder than retrospectively evaluating." Those who work in emergency services know very well what is meant by this statement. The present case shows how difficult it can be sometimes to make the "right" decision, as often one cannot be sure which one this is.

Half an hour before sunrise and thus before the official readiness for duty, the EMS control center calls the EMS helicopter station and asks if a mission on a country road about 18 flight minutes (approx. 45 km (28 miles) by air) away in the rural part of the EMS helicopter's area of operations would be possible. We, that is a police officer and pilot of the federal police, a rescue assistant of the professional fire brigade and I as an emergency physician of the professional fire brigade Duisburg / Germany, check the helicopter and 10 min later we take off with our "Christoph 9" into the morning and arrive at the scene of the accident at 6:50 am. Already on the approach we see the crashed car standing on a meadow in front of a tree; the fire brigade has already cut off the roof of the car and the first arriving emergency physician is trying to help the patient. We land on the meadow about 50 m (55 yards) next to the accident site and then report to the incident commander of the fire brigade and the emergency physician who is with the patient trapped in the vehicle. Based on accident witnesses, it turns out that the approximately 45-year-old patient drove her upper class car into a road tree at full speed and without braking; we cannot determine a cause of the accident. The front of the car has been so deformed by the accident that direct treatment of the patient without removing the roof was not possible. Between the accident and the removal of

F. Marx (✉)
Intensive Care Helicopter Christoph Giessen, Malteser Hilfsdienst Diözese Münster,
Giessen / Münster, Germany
e-mail: drmarx@web.de

V. Wenzel (ed.), *Case Studies in Emergency Medicine*,
https://doi.org/10.1007/978-3-662-67249-5_46

the roof, about 20 min passed; meanwhile, the rescue forces have been on site for about 35 min.

The engine room has pushed so deep into the passenger compartment that both lower legs are pressed and fractured under the front seat. The front seat is also raised cover-wise by the deformation of the passenger cell; as a result, the upper legs are only limitedly visible. The patient's respiration is bradypnoeic with a frequency of 8 breaths per minute, the airways are clear. Breathing is assisted with a mask and 100% oxygen and the cervical spine is immobilized. A carotid pulse is palpable, but not pulses on the upper arm and on the radial artery, which points to a severe shock state. The automatic blood pressure measurement does not produce a result; the manual measurement results in a systolic blood pressure of only 60 mmHg, since the use of the stethoscope is impossible due to the exterior noise from the power generator and the cutting device of the fire department as well as the noise of voices from the rescue workers. The patient is unconscious and reacts to strong pain stimuli with uncoordinated defense movements. Several puncture sites on the arms testify to the frustrated attempts of the first arriving rescue workers to create a venous access; I also cannot find a vein on the arm. My puncture attempt of the right internal jugular vein also runs—as expected—frustrated in the sitting patient. Therefore, I choose the method of intraosseous puncture of the humerus head with a drill, since the lower legs are not accessible to me as a preferred puncture site. The puncture succeeds easily and after functional control an infusion with hydroxyethyl starch 6% is connected; using the infusion pump, the infusion runs freely in the beam. The emergency physician quickly injects 2 ml of cafedrin / theodrenalin to raise blood pressure. However, this does not lead to a significant increase in systolic blood pressure within 3 min, which is checked closely by manual means. Therefore, we connect an infusion pump with norepinephrine (5 mg/50 ml with 15 ml/h). We measure blood pressure every minute while the fire department feverishly tries to free the patient's legs. As another 3 min later the blood pressure still does not rise, I double the speed of the norepinephrine infusion pump to 30 ml/h. Now, with an infusion volume of in the meantime 750 ml of hydroxyethyl starch, the blood pressure rises to 85 mmHg systolic.

Probably due to improved cerebral perfusion, the patient suddenly moves; in particular, she performs defensive movements with her arms, which in turn leads to dislocation of the intraosseous cannula. The infusion is then stopped and a new puncture is made in the area of the humerus head on the contralateral side. This is done without problems and both volume substitution and infusion of norepinephrine work smoothly. To avoid movements, the patient is now anesthetized with 0.2 mg fentanyl and 15 mg hypnomidate and subsequently paralyzed with 100 mg succinylcholine. The subsequent intubation attempt fails several times in the upright patient, so I decide to continue the ventilation manually with a breathing bag and the Esmarch-handle behind the patient. With sufficient spontaneous respiration, this synchronized intermittent ventilation with the self-inflatable bag works quite well for me. I hold the mask with both hands and a rescue assistant ventilates the patient with a tidal volume of about 400 ml. Another rescue assistant carefully ensures that the patient does not move her arm. As soon as the fire department arrived, they set up a number of halogen lamps to have enough working light in the dawn and to avoid hypothermia of the patient in view of the 5°C (41 °F) outside temperature. Finally, after 55 min, the patient is freed from the vehicle; in the ambulance, anesthesia is deepened and intubation is now successful. A naso-gastric tube is placed through the mouth, as air has entered the stomach during mask ventilation. Puncture attempts of the femoral vein and the left internal jugular vein fail; a puncture of the left subclavian vein is done without problems and further infusion solutions are now administered through this venous access. During inspection of the patient, it is now noticed that the right pupil is much wider than the left pupil and reacts slower to light. Both lower legs have open fractures in several places; the thorax and pelvis have no abnormalities. With a norepinephrine infusion of 3 mg/h, a systolic blood pressure of 80 mmHg is achieved; heart rate is 120/min. The patient is now transferred to the helicopter stretcher; we plan to fly to a university hospital that is only about 5 min away by helicopter. Treatment in the ambulance with venous access, anesthesia, intubation, examination and wound care takes about 20 min, so that now about 90 min have passed since the accident.

During the startup phase of the EMS helicopter, the patient suddenly has ventricular tachycardia, which progresses into ventricular fibrillation. The startup process is aborted and the engines are shut down. The patient is defibrillated with 200 J and we perform chest compressions. This leads to stabilization of the circulation within 2 min, which is recognizable by an increasing expiratory carbon dioxide. A blood pressure measurement on the upper arm does not result in anything. The patient is now transferred to the ambulance; due to the unstable circulation, transport by helicopter is no longer possible. When loading the patient into the ambulance, cardiac arrest occurs again. In the event of asystole, we now start chest compressions again and drive to a local hospital that is only 5 km (3 miles) away. Here an automatic device for chest compressions is connected; 30 min later, resuscitation efforts are discontinued. No autopsy was performed to determine the exact pattern of injury.

Discussion
There are many aspects to consider this mission as unusual. Especially in air rescue, the safety aspect is of great importance and therefore in critical situations such as darkness and bad weather, a mission is more likely to be rejected because of the associated risks, than it is carried out with high risk for the emergency personnel [1]. Registration for daily duty of the EMS helicopter at 07:00 AM is therefore also an established procedure, from which is only rarely deviated. However, the pilot estimated the light conditions at the expected time of arrival at the scene of the accident and that was the reason why he was willing to carry out this flight. While take-offs and landings at approved landing sites for helicopters are relatively safe even in darkness or twilight, this situation is completely different for external landings—too easily cables, wires or ground obstacles can be overlooked, which can then lead to fatal accidents [2]. In the USA, where EMS helicopter traditionally

fly during the day and at night, in 2008 the most dangerous profession was "pilot of an EMS helicopter", even before the traditionally very dangerous professions of deep-sea fishermen, coal miners and loggers. In fact, in 2008 in the USA, 29 people died in 12 accidents with EMS helicopters; so 2 fatal accidents occurred per 100,000 flight hours, while 1.3 fatal accidents occurred per 100,000 flight hours in general aviation and only 0.08 in commercial aviation.

It has been shown to be effective that the medical crew not only introduces themselves to the EMS colleagues at the accident site, but also to the fire department's incident commander, in order to coordinate the technical and medical rescue. After several attempts to rescue the trapped patient with rescue shears and a rescue spreader failed, we decided to pull the wrecked vehicle apart between 2 fire department vehicles about 45 min after the rescue effort began; a time period that often occurs for a difficult technical rescue [3, 4]. Finally, it was possible to pull the front vehicle far enough away from the front seats so that the patient could be lifted out of the vehicle sideways.

In the end, my decision to carry out a helicopter transport was questionable; perhaps the immediate transport to the smaller hospital nearby would have been more sensible, even though the resources there were scarce and a subsequent transfer would have been necessary after initial stabilization. This shows that a decision cannot be made categorically when it comes to the question "stay & play vs. load & go", but is strongly dependent on the situation, for example on blood loss, volume resuscitation and injury pattern [5]. The use of intraosseous needles in emergency medicine has experienced a renaissance in recent years [6]. Usually the anterior edge of the tibia is chosen because it is easy to identify and because fixation of the needle usually works safely; other puncture sites such as on the humerus as in our patient or on the radius are also possible, but are not used as often. In our case, intraosseous infusion was not sufficient to correct the volume deficit; it was also not possible to insert a central venous catheter in the car, probably because of the patient's sitting position with a severe volume deficit. It cannot be answered which outcome our patient would have had without the entrapment in the car; but the duration of the entrapment shows how fatal the time can be for the outcome in severe post-traumatic shock [7].

46.1 Conclusion

Despite very good cooperation between medical and technical personnel, it was initially not possible to rescue the trapped patient and then stabilize circulation. Given these frustrations and a subjectively felt helplessness, one must keep a cool head and be aware that one has to make decisions constantly during such a mission, even though one can only assess many unknown, indeed unpredictable variables to a limited extent. It is much more difficult to decide prospectively than to evaluate retrospectively.

References

1. Baker SP, Grabowski JG, Dodd RS, Shanahan DF, Lamb MW, Li GH (2006) EMS helicopter crashes: what influences fatal outcome? Ann Emerg Med 47:351–356
2. Hinkelbein J, Spelten O, Neuhaus C, Hinkelbein M, Ozgur E, Wetsch WA (2013) Injury severity and seating position in accidents with German EMS helicopters. Accid Anal Prev 59:283–288
3. Nutbeam T, Fenwick R, Hobson C, Holland V, Palmer M (2015) Extrication time prediction tool. Emerg Med J 32:401–403
4. Nutbeam T, Fenwick R, Hobson C, Holland V, Palmer M (2014) The stages of extrication: a prospective study. Emerg Med J 31:1006–1008
5. Wears RL, Winton CN (1990) Load and go versus stay and play: analysis of prehospital i. v. fluid therapy by computer simulation. Ann Emerg Med 19:163–168
6. Helm M, Schlechtriemen T, Haunstein B, Gassler M, Lampl L, Braun J (2013) Intraosseous infusion in the German Air Rescue Service: guideline recommendations versus mission reality. Anaesthesist 62:981–987
7. Demetriades D, Chan L, Cornwell E, Belzberg H, Berne TV, Asensio J, Chan D, Eckstein M, Alo K (1996) Paramedic vs private transportation of trauma patients. Effect on outcome. Arch Surg 131:133–138

Cardiologist with Heart Attack

47

Jan Breckwoldt

▶ What if physicians themselves become patients? How objectively can they assess their own illness? And how should colleagues behave correctly towards "physicians-patients"? The present case provides approaches to address these problems.

The mission statement is "severe chest pain" in a well-to-do inner-city area. At the mission address, we are let into a well-kept and elegantly furnished new building by the patient himself. The man in his mid-sixties has kept himself physically well, but shows the classic clinical signs of an acute coronary syndrome. We work through our routine for the treatment of an acute coronary syndrome quickly and while writing the 12-channel ECG, we quickly get into conversation with the patient. He retired half a year ago and has now moved to the city to enjoy the rich cultural offer. He was active as an interventional cardiologist until the end. Meanwhile, the ECG strip comes out of the machine and our joint visual diagnosis leaves no doubt about the ST-segment-elevation infarction. The patient has seen and treated such an ECG hundreds of times in his patients. With his symptomatology, he probably suspected something, but is nevertheless surprised that now the ECG strip clearly shows his own myocardial infarction. The work routine of our physician-manned ambulance now always includes the question of inclusion in the current myocardial infarction study, at that time a randomized, placebo-controlled comparison of a thrombolytic agent within the first 3 h of the myocardial infarction. The colleague refuses randomization. So we continue to treat him conventionally, with prior notice in the cardiac catheterization laboratory. When loading him into the ambulance, he suddenly develops ventricular fibrillation, but after two

J. Breckwoldt (✉)
University Hospital , Department of Anesthesiology, Zürich, Switzerland
e-mail: jan.breckwoldt@usz.ch

defibrillations including 2 min of chest compressions, he is rhythmologically and hemodynamically stable again. If he had not regained spontaneous circulation, we would have given him thrombolysis in accordance with the guidelines. The patient receives multiple stenting in the cardiac catheterization laboratory and recovers well.

Discussion

The treatment of physicians is a difficult field; British colleagues say about it: "With medics, things tend to go wrong"; US colleagues say: "Physicians are the worst patients". The fact that disproportionately many physicians do not have a family physician shows that many find it very difficult to take on the role of a patient, probably because they do not like to confront their own weakness. There is often an unspoken mistrust that adversely affects the quality of treatment [1]. Many doctors find it embarrassing to have to reveal their health concerns and needs, their self-diagnosis may be wrong or they may have existential fears if, for example, a depression or substance abuse spreads among colleagues perceived as competition [1]. Furthermore, there is often a professional skepticism towards treating physicians as well as fears that the confidentiality of information is endangered, as can be read from various reports on the treatment deficits in cases of illness [2]. In an English study, 84% of the drugs that they had taken in the last five years were self-prescribed by general practitioners [3]. When an external evaluation of the selection and dosage of the respective drugs was carried out, this self-medication was rated as wrong or insufficient in more than three quarters of the cases. "Illness does not belong to us", scientists from London titled their study in which they asked general practitioners about their own illness [4]; for example, a general practitioner with a psychiatric illness felt guilty of being ill and saw himself as a failure, two other general practitioners with a thyrotoxic crisis or hepatitis tried to significantly reduce the medically prescribed rest period. A researcher from Heidelberg / Germany describes the way physicians deal with their own illness as a development in five stages [5]. While in medical school, after learning about many diseases, a reactive hypochondria can develop, the "hard" medical phase follows with dogmatic health, which gladly represses disease signals. In the third phase, the physician does notice annoying complaints such as headaches or insomnia, but avoids consulting colleagues and prefers to treat himself. If, in the fourth phase, a symptom makes the physician objectively unable to work, he seeks collegial conversation, but remains inconsistent through "physician-shopping" and lack of follow-up, which ultimately makes him feel abandoned by himself. In the fifth phase, the physician is a suffering patient who seeks a compassionate treating physician who is also able to assert himself against him; only from here on are physicians normal patients [5]. These mechanisms should be made conscious and also discussed openly with "physician patients". Even if you maintain a professional distance, it can happen quickly that you omit certain diagnostic or therapeutic steps or implement them half-heartedly or too cautiously. In non-emergency situations, it is relatively easy to take a step back and pass the task on to more experienced colleagues or to emotionally less involved physicians. But this is not possible in the emergency medical service.

The head of the Institute for Medical Health in Villingen-Schwenningen / Germany describes ten recommendations for the "physician patient" [6], namely:

1. Seek help in time;
2. consult another physician, not yourself;
3. ask the treating physician to treat you as he would any other patient;
4. have a medical record made;
5. get all the recommendations that "normal" patients get;
6. follow the normal course of examination and treatment;
7. absolutely follow the recommendations (e.g. medication, diet, sick leave);
8. inform your family and friends;
9. also inform your colleagues and
10. reflect on your lifestyle in relation to your illness.

On the other hand, he also formulates ten recommendations for the physician treating a sick physician, [6] namely

1. thoroughly examine the "physician-patient";
2. pay attention to open and comprehensive communication;
3. clearly formulate what you think is the best treatment;
4. keep a medical record;
5. follow your usual routine (no exceptions, no short-cuts, no VIP bonus);
6. ensure the confidentiality of the data;
7. explain all recommendations thoroughly;
8. only you decide on the duration of the hospital treatment and sick leave;
9. You are the treating physician, your colleague the patient and
10. create a network in which physicians are treated well.

An emeritus neurologist from the University of Colorado comes to very similar recommendations from his 43 years of experience in treating physicians [7]:

Do not accept patients with special status, for whom you feel pressure or anxiety in their treatment;

- carry out the examination and treatment as usual;
- openly discuss the fears of the "physician-patient";
- define early and exactly your "physician-physician-patient" relationship;
- avoid excessive sympathy or empathy;
- discuss the planned diagnostics and treatment in detail to reduce anxiety;

- insist on enough time to discuss your opinion and recommendations well;
- discuss personal matters and ensure absolute confidentiality;
- proceed professionally and expect unjustified criticism as well.

47.1 Conclusion

From an emergency medical perspective, it is important to communicate openly as early as possible in the treatment of "doctor-patients", with regard to the patient's fears, one's own safety and insecurity, the diagnostic and therapeutic approach and absolute confidentiality. All processes should be carried out and documented as carefully as with all other patients in order to be able to act with sufficient professional distance.

References

1. Kay M, Mitchell G, Clavarino A, Doust J (2008) Doctors as patients: a systematic review of doctors' health access and the barriers they experience. Br J Gen Pract 58:501–508
2. Lam ST (2014) Special considerations in the care of the physician-patient: a lesson for medical education. Acad Psychiatry 38:632–637
3. Chambers R, Belcher J (1992) Self-reported health care over the past 10 years: a survey of general practitioners. Br J Gen Pract 42:153–156
4. McKevitt C, Morgan M (1997) Illness doesn't belong to us. J R Soc Med 90:491–495
5. Ripke T (2000) The sick physician: opportunity for a better understanding of the patient. Dtsch Ärzteblatt 97:A-237–240
6. Maulen B (2008) Physicians as patients–physicians treating other physicians. Dtsch Med Wochenschr 133:30–33
7. Schneck SA (1998) „Doctoring" doctors and their families. JAMA 280:2039–2042

Fall From Tree House

Peter Hilbert-Carius

▶ There are events that remain without words—like this one.

Felix is a happy, alert 9-year-old boy who plays on his small "tree house" on an August day at 1:30 pm. On this vacation day, Felix, his mother and his sister host a visit from a family friend and her daughter. Felix's father is working as an emergency physician on an EMS helicopter that day, so he is not at home. Since "tree houses" are more for boys, Felix's sister and her friend decide to go to the pool and Felix plays by himself on his house. Here he has a small pulley and a plate swing, the rope of which he has wrapped around the railing of the "tree house".

How exactly it happens, nobody can say, since the event happens unobserved. Somehow the little Felix must have lost his balance and falls from about 1.5 m from the platform of his "tree house". In doing so, he must have come across the neck on the rope of his swing plate in the fall. After the fall on the lawn, Felix gets up again and wants to walk towards the house. Since the family's friend has noticed that Felix has landed on the lawn, she runs in his direction to see if he has hurt himself. Felix takes 3 steps in her direction and expresses with hardly audible voice that he could not get any air. Then he becomes unconscious and collapses. From his mouth runs some bloody-foamy secretion. The family's friend, who hurries to Felix, is a trained nurse and recognizes the drama of the situation. Due to the unconsciousness and the lack of breathing, she begins to revive the little Felix. In parallel, the emergency call is made at 13:47 at the responsible EMS control center. At 13:49 the physicain-manned ambulance and the ambulance alarmed leave and reach the scene of the accident at 13:52. Here Felix is still being

P. Hilbert-Carius (✉)
Department of Anesthesiology, Intensive Care, and Emergency Medicine,
BG Trauma Hospital Bergmannstrost, Halle / Saale, Germany
e-mail: Dr.PeterHilbert@web.de

V. Wenzel (ed.), *Case Studies in Emergency Medicine*,
https://doi.org/10.1007/978-3-662-67249-5_48

resuscitated; the EMS team takes over the resuscitation attempt and continues it. After connecting the monitoring, a bradycardia with 30/min and a peripheral oxygen saturation of 84% is shown in the monitoring device. To secure the airway, Felix is intubated by the emergency physician, which apparently succeeds without problems, with a lot of blood in the pharynx and larynx. When trying to ventilate via the endotracheal tube, it becomes clear that the lungs are not being inflated on both sides and with each attempt to breathe, a skin emphysema develops on the neck. In parallel to the attempt to secure the airway, a venous access is inserted in the right elbow. Due to the impossibility of ventilating via the endotracheal tube, this is removed again and the CPR attempt is continued with bag-valve-mask ventilation. It quickly becomes clear that there must be a respiratory problem that is difficult to treat prehospitally. The attempt at a surgical airway is omitted. Due to the proximity to a hospital of maximum care, the decision is made to take Felix to the hospital with ongoing CPR. At 14:07, about 20 min after the emergency call, the transport is carried out with ongoing CPR. During the prehospital therapy interval, Felix receives a total of 3 times 0.3 mg ($= 300\ \mu g$) epinephrine. At 14:09 the team reaches the emergency room of the hospital informed in advance. Here in the ECG already an asystole is present.

In the emergency room, the colleagues from ENT first try to intubate Felix by means of a rigid bronchoscope, which, however, leads to the same frustrated result as the intubation attempt by the emergency physician and does not contribute to secure the airway. Despite ongoing resuscitation measures and injection of epinephrine, asystole is still present in the ECG, which is not surprising, since a minimum of oxygen is necessary for successful resuscitation of a child's heart, which has not yet reached the child's lungs at this point in time. Due to the frustrated intubation attempts by means of a rigid bronchoscope, the decision is now made to carry out an emergency tracheotomy. This is made more difficult by the massive skin emphysema, but is successful. Even after it has now been possible to secure the airway and oxygenate the child, all further resuscitation measures remain unsuccessful. The ECMO set up in the meantime is also not used and little Felix finally dies due to hypoxia that cannot be eliminated in time. The forensic examination shows that Felix was actually a healthy boy who finally died of severe hypoxia when the trachea was torn off 4 cm above the carina.

Discussion

Traumatic tracheal injuries or tears are extremely rare, rarer than iatrogenic injuries to the trachea [1], but life-threatening. Many of these traumatic tracheobronchial injuries end up fatal outside of the hospital and only a high level of attention can already raise the suspicion prehospitally of these injury patterns [2]. Clinical signs that may suggest the presence of a tracheobronchial injury after an appropriate trauma include dyspnoea, cyanosis, haemoptysis, dysphonia/hoarseness, skin emphysema, persistent pneumothorax, hypotension up to cardiac arrest [1, 3, 4]. Prehospital diagnosis is extremely difficult and the definitive diagnosis is usually only made in the hospital. In addition to radiological methods, such as chest x-ray or appropriate computed tomography, which usually only provide indirect evidence of the injury, endoscopic methods are available with which the injury can be visualized itself. A relatively new method is multi-planar 3-D reconstruction using multi-slice computed tomography, which allows virtual bronchoscopy []2]. In addition to the possible difficulties in prehospital diagnosis, the prehospital therapy can be very difficult. The acute treatment begins, as with any trauma, according to the ABCDE rules of PHTLS®/ATLS®. Securing of oxygenation has the highest priority. Therefore, (if not even should) in spontaneously breathing patients with good oxygenation, intubation should be avoided as far as possible, because an imprudent anesthesia induction and intubation can lead to the following problems in a so far possibly still sufficiently breathing patient: In the context of rapid sequence induction, problems may develop with upper airway injuries resulting in difficulties in intubation up to a complete laceration of the airway with its deleterious consequences and in the context of paralysis, a loss of muscle tone can lead to an airway obstruction, up to all catastrophic consequences [2, 5]. With increasing dyspnea, disturbed breathing and oxygenation, intubation at the emergency site is however life-saving, because by increasing swelling, bleeding or skin and mediastinal emphysema, endotracheal intubation may eventually become impossible. If, as in the described case, oral intubation or ventilation via the endotracheal tube is not possible, a tracheotomy or open tracheotomy may be necessary at the emergency site [4]. In the described case, this procedure could possibly have been life-saving, but this assumption remains purely speculative. In dramatic situations, as they presented themselves in the case of Felix, often only invasive "dramatic" treatment options can yield the desired success. The basis for this is a mastery of appropriate therapeutic measures. Therefore, at this point, only every person working in emergency medicine can be advised to intensively deal with invasive emergency measures in the course of their training and to practice them accordingly [6]. The actual emergency itself is the worst time for this. Another possible option at the moment when it was clear that ventilation via the endotracheal tube was not possible, would have been a battery-operated flexible bronchoscope. Perhaps one could have seen the distal tracheal opening at the end of the tube and then placed the tube under control by carefully withdrawing it. Unfortunately, such bronchoscopes are only sporadically available on physician-manned EMS vehicles [7, 8].

Conclusion above is lacking had to die with his young 9 years due to an A-problem (airway) according to PHTLS®/ATLS®, because it was not possible to treat this problem adequately outside of or inside the hospital in a timely manner. A-problems have the highest treatment priority according to PHTLS®/ATLS®, as the case shows in a sad and dramatic way impressively. Furthermore, the case should remind us that all those working in prehospital and clinical intramural medicine should intensively deal with the management of A-, B-, C-, D-, E-problems.

48.1 Last Words

In memory of Felix (* 17.03.2005 – † 11.08.2014), who was actually born to live, but had no luck. The parents of Felix have expressly agreed to this publication in the hope that this case discussion may be helpful in similar emergencies.

"It is hard for me to live without you, to give everything at any time every day. I often think back to what was, to every so beloved past day.

I imagine that you are standing next to me and that you are accompanying me on every one of my ways. I think of so much since you are no longer there, because you showed me how valuable life is.

We were born to live, with the wonders of each time, never to forget each other for eternity. We were born to live for the one moment, because each one of us felt how valuable life is.

It still hurts to create new space, to let something new in with a good feeling. At this moment you are close to me again, as on every so beloved past day.

It is my wish to allow dreams again, to look forward to the future without regret. I see a meaning since you are no longer there, because you showed me how valuable my life is [9]."

References

1. Paraschiv M (2014) Iatrogenic tracheobronchial rupture. J Med. Life 3:343–348
2. Prokakis C, Koletsis EN, Dedeilias P, Fligou F, Filos K, Dougenis D (2014) Airway trauma: a review on epidemiology, mechanisms of injury, diagnosis and treatment. J Cardiothorac Surg 9:117
3. Palade E, Passlick B (2011) Surgery of traumatic tracheal and tracheobronchial injuries. Chirurg 82:141–147
4. Welter S, Hoffmann H (2013) Injuries to the tracheo-bronchial tree. Zentralbl Chir 138:111–116
5. Abernathy JH III, Reeves ST (2010) Airway catastrophes. Curr Opin Anaesthesiol 23:41–46
6. Zink W, Volkl A, Martin E, Gries A (2002) Invasive emergency techniques (INTECH). A training concept in emergency medicine. Anaesthesist 51:853–862
7. Thierbach A, Lipp M (1999) Fiberoptic intubation in an emergency. Notfall Rettungsmed 2:105–110
8. Wagner MP (1999) Fiberoptic intubation in an emergency. Notfall Rettungsmed 2:39–47
9. The Duke and Unholy. Born to live. Unholy. 29–1–2010. Vertigo Berlin. Ref Type: Sound Recording

Thrombolysis

49

Franziska Böhler

I had thrown my notice of termination in the mailbox of my nursing manager. After 13 years in the intensive care unit, many weekends and two children who could only experience their parents together once a month, it was time for a change. Late shift on Friday: The feeling of only working here for six more months was strange, but I decided to suppress the pain of separation. During the handover, I was assigned two monitoring patients and a critical case. The critical patient had undergone major abdominal surgery the day before and had already complained of shortness of breath to the colleagues in the early shift. When I entered the room, the approximately 50-year-old man was already sitting upright in bed, sweating and gasping for air. Within minutes, his condition deteriorated dramatically and we had to start resuscitation.

When the diagnosis pulmonary embolism was made, a decision had to be made together with the surgeons, we decided to carry out a thrombolysis. In the meantime, the man's wife and two adult daughters were also informed about the situation. I can understand from my own painful experience how devastating such news can feel. In the stressful everyday work life, one sometimes forgets in which extreme situations the relatives are when they see a loved one in the middle of a highly technologized room on the intensive care unit, surrounded by machinery and cables, have to give up control and experience a possibly life-threatening situation. And above all: Can't do anything yourself but wait.

F. Böhler (✉)
Emma Hospital, Department of Anesthesiology, Seligenstadt, Germany
e-mail: Franzi.Pfeifer@gmx.de

V. Wenzel (ed.), *Case Studies in Emergency Medicine*,
https://doi.org/10.1007/978-3-662-67249-5_49

In a short stable interval, we let the relatives into the room. While the man's wife calmly took his hand, the oldest daughter collapsed crying at the bed. I don't have to say that the human component is actually nothing that you could prioritize—but if there are two other patients to take care of, then there is actually nothing left to do. In a short conversation, I tried to describe the patient's condition, but had to send the family away again because the patient became bradycardic again. In the meantime, the surgical colleagues had decided on an abdominal CT to detect any perfusion problems. Due to the thrombolysis, the patient was now bleeding from the bladder, nose, mouth and the surgical wound on the stomach. The resident physician and I had a bad feeling about the thought of transport to the CT over two floors, especially since the patient was highly catecholamine-dependent and unstable. So I got the portable ventilator and started to rebuild all connections and disconnections. Then we went.

We passed the exit door of our intensive care unit and brushed over a small floor wave, so that the bed wobbled a little—the blood pressure dropped sharply due to the minimal vibration. The elevator was already there, we drove in carefully and chose the second floor, where the CT was located. The patient suddenly became maximally circulatory unstable; the elevator door opened and the monitor confirmed asystole. So we drove quickly to the CT corridor and started resuscitating again. While the resident physician ordered reinforcements by phone, I carried out the thoracic compressions. The man was losing more and more blood, with each thoracic compression I could literally see the blood dripping from the wound. Meanwhile, a colleague and the senior physician had arrived to stabilize the patient primarily on the corridor. We ordered more blood transfusions, opened the emergency kit and finally stood in a huge pool of blood.

While eight hands tried to generate a stable circulation again, I heard the elevator going down. It stopped two floors later, someone got on, and the elevator came back. The doors opened and in front of us were the relatives of the patient. Since the CT would take a while, they had decided to get some fresh air, the exit was on the same floor. The sight that greeted them should not be experienced by any relative: four hospital employees, who were busy drawing up syringes, injecting drugs, turning on the ventilator, still resuscitating—and everything, really everything, full of blood. Both daughters collapsed screaming at that moment. The despair and the pain that came with it burned persistently in me. The man who happened to be in the elevator with us pressed the button back to the ground floor. After what felt like an eternity, we stabilized the patient and could start the journey back to the intensive care unit. The relatives had meanwhile returned to the waiting area, from there you could see the corridor on which we drove past with the patients. Again the children broke into tears, screamed, cried and loudly called "Papa!", "Papa!"

Back on the ward, my resident physician decided to insert a Shaldon catheter for dialysis and volume replacement. In the meantime, my colleagues had taken care of the other two patients who had been assigned to me. After the creation of two large-lumen intravenous lines, we also started with hemofiltration. It didn't look good. After a few years of work, after so many patients, you get a feeling for some courses. We were all sure that day or at the latest that night our patient would not survive this day.

I asked the relatives who had been waiting all day to come back to the room in the evening. I had removed the (blood) traces of thrombolysis as best I could; the patient seemed stable for a short time. I was tired. After this shift, it was not just the eight hours I had been on my feet non-stop—I was also psychologically exhausted. This extreme situation in which the family was—which they carried to the outside, in which they tried to find comfort with me, weighed me down at the end of the shift. Also because I was sure that this man would not survive the night. And that made me feel so incredibly sorry. When I came back for the late shift the next day, my eyes quickly fell on the transfer sheet—the patient was alive. Since I only came on duty every other weekend due to my part-time job, I could not observe the course of this patient on a daily basis. After a few weeks, shortly before Christmas, the patient was tracheotomized and planned for a rehabilitation hospital. The first attempts with the speech cannula were sufficient.

After some time had passed, I received an invitation: The family had organized a party. Among the guests were, among others, the visceral surgeon who had spoken out in favor of thrombolysis at the time, the resident physician who resuscitated with me on the CT corridor—and me. I had always tried to maintain professional distance in dealing with patients, but this case had come so close to me that I gladly accepted the invitation. In my last memory there was a weakened man, slightly icteric and still tracheotomized in a white hospital bed. Nine months later, the same person suddenly stood in front of me—with a broad grin on his face and a beer in his hand.

Discussion

A family member in an intensive care unit is the maximum stress for relatives for a variety of reasons; the most important are probably the difficulty of understanding the situation, the powerlessness of almost nothing to do and of course the fear that the illness or injury is fatal. In Pittsburgh, Pennsylvania, 24 family members were interviewed about a month after the death of a relative in an intensive care unit in a structured interview. All of them experienced the inclusion in the therapy decision as valuable, because in this way helplessness was reduced and a piece of control over the situation was regained, and human suffering was reduced [1]. Pediatricians in Miami, Florida, interviewed the parents half a year after the death of 47 infants or children in an intensive care unit about what helped the least and the most [2]. Compassion, sensitivity, willingness to help, experience, competence, understandable explanations as well as the inclusion of parents in therapy and decision-making were perceived as positive. The parents saw the most negative conflicts with the intensive care unit team (e.g. "I explained that to you yesterday—didn't you understand it?") as well as insensitive communication (e.g. "Your son had an accident. Are you willing to donate organs?"). In a Norwegian study, the satisfaction with the intensive care unit team understandably correlated with a good outcome; but also with good, consistent information about the patient's condition [3]. In Paris, the relatives, the patient *and* the intensive care unit team make daily notes in a diary, which has improved the mutual understanding, trust and information within the family of relatives, but also of the intensive care unit team in a very impressive way [4]. Such an exchange can be very intense and fulfilling; a colleague told me a similar story to the one above about a roaring celebration of life with all relatives when a patient could be discharged home after a long complicated intensive care stay.

49.1 Conclusion

Sometimes—possibly even too often—we exclude or neglect relatives in our work. This is usually not done with bad intentions, especially in times of nursing shortages, it is also a question of resources: If there is already no time for patients to receive attention and care, then there is even less time for relatives. On the other hand, sometimes we may also not think enough about how our actions, our communication, our handling of situations shapes the experience of relatives. I admit that I had to stand on the other side myself—as a worried, hopeful, desperate relative—until I realized how crucial a caring approach to relatives can be. Relatives look closely at how we—the medical and nursing staff—behave: how we speak, how we react to situations and questions—and it affects them. Whether we have the extra few minutes or even ask how the relatives are doing themselves. Just how a sentence like "Visiting hours are now over." is formulated and pronounced—matter-of-factly or regretfully—can make a difference as to whether a relative grieves for a long time or leaves the ward with the feeling that a close person is in good hands.

In acute situations, things often have to happen very quickly, relatives have to be quickly removed from the room and sit stunned during a resuscitation attempt nearby. This can usually not be avoided in the current situation, but it is important what happens afterwards: That we take the time to explain what happened, show empathy, possibly express sincere regret. And in the event of a death, to give the relatives plenty of time to say goodbye [5] is often quickly sidelined in the hospital. All the more it is appreciated if attention is paid to it.

The case described above is extreme and I know that the relatives of the affected patient were in psychological care to process the experience—such an emergency measure can shake outsiders that much. We should therefore never forget to always keep the perspective of the relatives in mind in our work and—to the extent that resources permit—to take them into account and show empathy. Because I can assure you from my own experience: When working through painful processes, this can be relevant, decisive or at least helpful.

References

1. Nunez ER, Schenker Y, Joel ID, Reynolds CF 3rd, Dew MA, Arnold RM, Barnato AE (2015) Acutely bereaved surrogates' stories about the decision to limit life support in the ICU. Crit Care Med 43:2387–2393
2. Brooten D, Youngblut JM, Seagrave L, Caicedo C, Hawthorne D, Hidalgo I, Roche R (2013) Parent's perceptions of health care providers actions around child ICU death: what helped, what did not. Am J Hosp Palliat Care 30:40–49
3. Haave RO, Bakke HH, Schröder A (2021) Family satisfaction in the intensive care unit, a cross-sectional study from Norway. BMC Emerg Med 21:20
4. Garrouste-Orgeas M, Périer A, Mouricou P, Grégoire C, Bruel C, Brochon S, Philippart F, Max A, Misset B (2014) Writing in and reading ICU diaries: qualitative study of families' experience in the ICU. PLoS One 9:e110146.
5. Böhler F, Kubsova J (Hrsg) (2020) I'm a nurse: Warum ich meinen Beruf als Krankenschwester liebe- trotz allem. Heyne, München.

Bernd Fertig

In August, at noon, a call for help comes in to the EMS helicopter in Lima, Peru, from the Swiss embassy regarding a mountaineer who, at a distance of approximately 450 km / 280 miles and an altitude of approximately 4600 m / 15100 feet, is suffering from altitude sickness. Due to the great distance, the Bell-212 helicopter is filled to capacity with fuel and three additional barrels (each 200 l) of jet fuel A1 are loaded. We unload the gasoline barrels at a distance of approximately 60 km (38 miles) from the site of operation. The co-pilot also remains there because the site of operation would be near the service peak altitude of approximately 5500 m / 18000 feet of the helicopter. Any, even seemingly minor, weight savings are helpful because, due to the decreasing air density, both the performance of the engines and the overall lift decrease and the helicopter must have power reserves just above ground level in order to avoid being brought down by strong winds in the mountains. After landing at the base camp, we learn that it is not a case of altitude sickness, but of an injured person who is approximately 5000 m / 16400 feet above sea level. At an outside temperature of −15 °C (5 °F), we find there, in a tent, a young, somnolent man (Glasgow Coma Scale 6) with regular, uncoordinated stretching and bending reactions on the left side of his body. The right pupil is dilated. The breathing is partly obstructed by the tongue with a breathing rate of 6/min; heart rate is 135/min, oxygen saturation 84% and blood pressure 110/80 mmHg. At an altitude of 5000 m / 16400 feet, such an oxygen saturation is normal, but it also only represents an arterial oxygen partial pressure of approximately 50 instead of approximately 95 mmHg at sea level [1], which

B. Fertig (✉)

Department of Paramedicine, University of San Marcos, Lima, Peru; and Autonomous University Gabriel Renè Moreno, Santa Cruz, Bolivia, Institute for Patient Safety and Quality in Emergency Medicine, Waldbronn, Germany

e-mail: bernd1003@hotmail.com

V. Wenzel (ed.), *Case Studies in Emergency Medicine*,
https://doi.org/10.1007/978-3-662-67249-5_50

is unfavorable in the case of a head injury. The injured person was hit on the head and right arm by an ice avalanche at an altitude of approximately 5900 m / 19350 feet while climbing to the summit in the afternoon of the day before and, as a result, suffered a head injury and a fracture of the forearm; subsequently, the increasingly disoriented mountaineer managed to descend, first with his climbing partner and then with the help of other climbers, to the base camp, which, however, took approximately 9 h for 900 altitude meters or 2950 feet. Later that morning, a high-altitude worker reaches the next village in 3 h instead of the usual 6 h, so that the first call for help comes in about 18 h after the accident. Due to the time pressure caused by bad weather, we can only provide a short initial treatment with oxygen inhalation, intravenous access and immobilization. We then fly to the intermediate landing site at an altitude of approximately 3000 m / 9800 feet, where our co-pilot and our gasoline barrels are waiting for us. The pilots fill the 600 L (158 gallons) of jet fuel A1 that has been prepared, we intubate the patient and can take off for the 90-minute flight to Lima about 24 h after the accident. This is followed by another 90 min in the ambulance between the airport and the hospital in this metropolis of 11 million inhabitants. After admission to the hospital, the patient undergoes immediately a craniotomy, during which an epidural hematoma is relieved. The patient is then quickly weaned and successfully extubated. He recovers very well, so that he can return to his Swiss home one week later by a normal airliner. After our return from Peru, we visit the patient on his mountain farm in Switzerland. It is a very moving reunion, because it has become clear to both our patient and the parents how much luck and good will of all involved had worked together here. This visit is also very special for us, because everything had a good ending- often the efforts had been similar in other missions, but the outcome was fatal for the patient. We sit for a long time with the whole family in front of the farm and enjoy the magnificent view over the mountains of the Swiss Alps. We are all aware that here it will hardly take 15 minutes for an EMS helicopter to arrive, while in Peru it takes many hours or even days for such a mission to clear the bureaucratic hurdles and for help to finally arrive.

Diskussion

The clinical development in this case is classic- after the trauma follows a "free interval" in which the climber was initially even able to descend independently, but then increasingly needed more help and showed the usual symptoms of an intracranial pressure increase with headache, vigilance disturbance, ipsilateral midriasis, and peripheral motor phenomena at base camp. If left untreated, the rising intracranial pressure causes a respiratory disturbance, which in turn, through hypoxia and hypercapnia, sets in motion an untreated lethal intracranial pressure vicious circle; in 1927, a mortality rate of 86% was described for this mechanism without therapy. [2]. In a study from Berlin, patients with a traumatic epidural hematoma and an initial Glasgow Coma Scale < 9 had a mortality of 15%, but the prehospital time was usually < 1 h and not 24 h as in our case. [3] It is almost impossible to find literature on such delayed urgent craniotomy because in industrialized countries, even if there is a time delay, such a procedure is usually started no later than 2.5 h after hospital admission-including about 1 h of prehospital time, i.e., about 3.5 h after the accident. [4].

For European mountaineers, a professional (air) EMS service and excellent hospital care are a matter of course. It always amazes me that tourists or mountaineers travelling to the mountains of the world also consider this to be self-evident in distant places. A foreign health insurance policy in one's pocket is a deceptive security, because the insured benefits on site are often simply not available. In the Andes of Peru, there is hardly any mobile phone network in most regions, so an emergency call without a satellite phone, as in our case, has to be made by a local "running messenger" who ran 20 km / 12 miles through valleys and over two passes to alert the EMS. The rescuers are often on foot themselves, which can take up to two weeks in some regions, and they also have hardly any medical equipment that would be comparable to a European mountain rescue service. The rescuers repeatedly experience the tragic experience that accident victims die from the consequences of long-term exposure to altitude, blood loss and shock, as well as inevitable hypothermia, even before their rescue, because the time interval between the accident and the arrival of the rescuers was several days. The availability of the EMS helicopter and relatively good weather in this case were also fortunate circumstances. Unfortunately, a nationwide primary air rescue service for everyone was not a matter of course in Peru at that time. The rule is a time-consuming organization of cost-sharing declarations. Overall, our injured mountaineer therefore had enormous luck—a single gap in the rescue chain, such as the lack of numerous rescuers in the high mountains or too bad flying weather, would probably have cost him his life.

In Peru, there are only one tenth of the cars in comparison to Germany, but in 2018 in Peru 19 times as many children under 15 died in road traffic accidents in relation to Germany. For adults, it is "only" the approximately threefold higher number of fatal traffic victims [5]. In Peru, there are about two accidents per year that are unimaginable in Germany, such as the crash of a tourist bus over an 80 m / 262 feet high cliff, in which 48 of the 57 bus passengers were immediately killed and four more died in hospital [6]. In 2018 alone, there were 5966 accidents involving buses in Peru, resulting in 38,323 injuries and 771 deaths [7]. There is a seat belt law, speed limits, a ban on alcohol at the wheel, a helmet requirement for motorcycle riders and a ban on mobile phones while driving in Peru, just as in Europe, but hardly anyone adheres to them. And if offences are punished by the police, this is usually done by a "tip" in the policeman's pocket. In Peru, the EMS reaches the accident site in 5% of cases in cities within 10 min and in 95% of cases within 20–30 min; in remote rural areas between 60 min and 4 h or even longer. Since mainly young people die in traffic accidents, the economic damage is enormous. A professional EMS could therefore save many lives with little investment.

Due to the long distances, poor roads and terrestrial obstacles, a supply of Peru with an exclusively ground-based EMS service is probably not feasible or affordable, while an air rescue service with extended aid deadlines of about 60 min in combination with some EMS vehicles can cover an extremely large area with a radius of about 220 km / 137 miles [2], which would correspond to more than the area of the state of Baden-Württemberg in Germany with 35751 km^2 (13804 square miles) area and 11.3 million population. This too may hardly be imaginable in Germany, but Peru is about 3.5 times larger than Germany with comparatively very difficult traffic infrastructure and partly sparsely populated regions in the mountains and the rainforest region. In the final development stage, it is planned to supply Peru with 20 EMS helicopters operated by the Peruvian Air Force. This would be a huge development step for Peruvian emergency medicine, even if this would also not be imaginable in comparison to Germany, since then Germany as a whole would be supplied with only six EMS helicopters and not with about 89 as is currently the case.

Until 2020 there was no air rescue system and no central EMS control centre in Peru; we are currently building this up with the support of the German federal government. The state-based ground EMS system "SAMU" (Servicio de Atención Médica de Urgencia) is organised as a rendezvous system after the German model. We have compiled this vision in an expert opinion for the Peruvian Ministry of Health in 2019. In 2021, in cooperation with Bolivia and Colombia, we will start a dual bachelor's degree programme at the Faculty of Medicine of the University of San Marcos according to the German curriculum of the emergency medical technician. Thus, our experience in the care of over 2600 emergency patients in the years 2000 to 2020 now leads to a re-organisation of the EMS in Peru, which we have always considered to be the basic health service for the entire population. The Peruvian policy intends to offer the EMS free of charge.

50.1 Conclusion

Rescuing a mountaineer who has had an accident at an altitude of 5000 m / 16400 feet in the Andes is possible, but in addition to the usual components of personal training, experience and technical aids, it takes insane luck to have all of this available without gaps and ad hoc. To implement an air rescue in Peru, we have invested almost 20 years of hard work to convince all parties of the sense, affordability and feasibility.

References

1. Imray C, Wright A, Subudhi A, Roach R (2010) Acute mountain sickness: pathophysiology, prevention, and treatment. Prog Cardiovasc Dis 52:467–484
2. Maugeri R, Anderson DG, Graziano F, Meccio F, Visocchi M, Iacopino DG. 2015 Conservative vs. surgical management of post-traumatic epidural hematoma: A case and review of literature. Am J Case Rep 16:811–817
3. Gutowski P, Meier U, Rohde V, Lemcke J, von der Brelie C (2018) Clinical outcome of epidural hematoma treated surgically in the era of modern resuscitation and trauma care world Neurosurg 118:e166–e174
4. Marcoux J, Bracco D, Saluja RS (2016) Temporal delays in trauma craniotomies. J Neurosurg 125:642–647
5. https://www.who.int/publications/i/item/9789241565684
6. https://www.zeit.de/gesellschaft/zeitgeschehen/2018-01/peru-verkehrsunfall-bus-strand-tote?utm_referrer=https%3A%2F%2F
7. https://andina.pe/agencia/noticia-accidentes-transito-dejan-771-muertos-el-pais-lo-va-del-2018-731877.aspx

Hyperventilation

51

Björn Hossfeld

We do our work in the emergency medical services with passion and concern for the patients entrusted to us, but at the end of the day we would rather report on the spectacular experiences. According to the slogan *"Triple-T"* it is of course great if we have been able to provide a severely injured patient with *a tube* and *two thoracic drains* in a time-critical manner before hospitalization and have handed him over stable in the emergency room. However, the less spectacular scene calls are not necessarily less challenging, or less exciting.

With the alarm keyword "Hyperventilation" on the pager we were on our way to a 14-year-old boy in a school and accordingly we joked on the way: "Again a Triple-T*: Talk-down (calm down verbally), Bag (in German: "Tüte" for rebreathing in hyperventilation) and Tavor® (pharmacologically calm*; in this case with lorazepam)". After all, acute hyperventilation syndrome is a common disorder, especially in young people, which rarely causes us diagnostic or therapeutic problems. Although in our perception young women have to be (not) medically treated more often, epidemiological studies show that the frequency is equally distributed between the two genders.

Situations in which strong affects such as fear are suppressed (for example, before difficult school tasks) are often the trigger for a hyperventilation syndrome in school age, which is characterized by paroxysmal, accelerated and deepened breathing. This in turn causes a reduction of dissolved carbon dioxide in the blood and as a consequence an increase in pH in the sense of a respiratory alkalosis. This pH increase in turn leads to a reduction of free calcium in the blood with the typical tetanic symptoms, such as paresthesia and paws position. These

B. Hossfeld (✉)
Department of Anesthesiology, Intensive Care, Emergency Medicine, and Pain Therapy, Federal Armed Forces Hospital, Ulm, Germany
e-mail: bjoern.hossfeld@uni-ulm.de

V. Wenzel (ed.), *Case Studies in Emergency Medicine*,
https://doi.org/10.1007/978-3-662-67249-5_51

somatic symptoms can intensify the patient's fear, triggering a further deepening of breathing and thus a circulus vitiosus. The rebreathing from a bag held in front of the patient's mouth and nose seems to be a logical consequence in order to make the carbon dioxide in the blood rise again, but is controversial because also cases of unnoticed hypoxia are described when employing this method. In a case series from San Francisco with supposed hyperventilation syndrome, a rebreathing therapy was applied but it was overlooked that the main pathophysiology was hypoxia or myocardial ischemia; all three patients died from this treatment error [1]. Therefore, monitoring of peripheral oxygen saturation is essential and an additional monitoring of end-tidal carbon dioxide can be extremely helpful.

I often find myself thinking that many ambulance calls could be handled just as well by a good EMS team without an EMS physician, usually faster and without any disadvantage for the patient. So on the way to this call, I also doubted the usefulness of my alarm. But on site the following situation presented itself. A 14-year-old male student was lying on a stretcher in the school's infirmary. The initial treatment was being carried out by the team of an ambulance, which by chance happened to be nearby and was the first vehicle to be alerted by the EMS control center. The patient had a clearly increased respiratory rate of over 30/min, which was impressively visible in the movements of a plastic bag held up. I was greeted with the words: "Sorry Doc, we can't do it without sedation." At first glance, the patient was unconscious. However, that this did not fit into the history of a classical hyperventilation syndrome had escaped the young ambulance crew; here, another cause for the tachypnoea had to be present. We established the intravenous access prepared for sedation. The blood sugar test carried out immediately from this showed a pronounced hyperglycaemia of >600 mg/dl. The high respiratory rate of the patient was therefore not due to a psychological stress reaction, but corresponded to the physiological reaction of the body, which was caused by the hyperglycaemic metabolism to compensate for ketoacidosis respiratorily. Accordingly, we infused generous amounts of cristalloid fluids, replaced the bag with an oxygen mask, and established end-tidal carbon dioxide measurement in addition to pulse oximetry, for which the measuring line was simply placed next to the mouth and nose under the oxygen mask thanks to the sidestream technology. This showed a value of 7 mmHg instead of the usual about 40 mmHg. The history did not reveal any previously known diabetes mellitus, so the patient was presented to the emergency room with suspicion of the first manifestation of a Type I diabetes. This diagnosis was confirmed.

Discussion

A fixation error is perhaps something deeply human because we usually professionally as well as personally welcome it when we encounter something familiar again and thus seemingly follow accustomed paths during an initial examination of a matter, even though they may be wrong or even are. A very nice example was described from Bonn: A man with signs of self-injury sat naked on a chair for 9 h in a neglected apartment, antipsychotic medications were lying on the dining table and the concerned neighbors said that "the man was known in the psychiatric facility" and had become increasingly conspicuous, e.g. by persecution mania and boards nailed to the door [2]. The emergency physician tried to get an overview but then ran out of time due to the request for a follow-up scene call. So what could be more natural than to transport this patient to the hospital in an ambulance and present him to a psychiatrist? However, the patient then became cardiorespiratory unstable, had to be intubated in the end and was finally operated on for a gastric perforation and four-quadrant peritonitis. A coronary intervention was also performed during the course. The initial symptomatology was therefore most likely due to a septic encephalopathy.

The hyperventilation syndrome is a differential diagnosis: Before we "impute" a mental diagnosis to a patient, we must clarify vital threatening causes of tachypnea [3]. The respiratory compensation of a metabolic acidosis is in the foreground, but other causes are also conceivable for a tachypnea. I remember, for example, a spontaneous pneumothorax in a young football player without trauma. In such cases, in addition to a careful past medical history, the appropriate experience and the clinical training of the emergency physician are extremely helpful. It is not about blaming the young paramedics of the ambulance being responsible. The pre-hospital conditions and the often time-critical action offer a certain risk for so-called "fixation errors". The fixation refers to the unhelpful trust in experiences from already experienced situations, which are similar to the current situation, but ultimately not the same. So if we focus on an aspect that we recognize—in the described case the tachypnea—and do not recognize the relevant difference to previously made experiences—namely that the patient is unconscious—then our experiences will lead us into a dead end. In the case example, this perception is further reinforced by apparently typical environmental conditions (young patient in a school), as in our memory the last hyperventilation syndromes have just occurred in this context. If we do not recognize the error in our assumption by mentally taking a step to the side and questioning the situation, we will not develop an idea for an alternative approach. Evie Fioratou and colleagues deal with this problem in their really worth reading study [4].

Fixation errors should be kept as low as possible using so-called Standard Operating Procedures (SOPs). While such SOPs can often be well represented as flowcharts, they often start from a suspected diagnosis or symptom. The case described shows that the clinical experience of the emergency physician is an essential component for the most likely suspected diagnosis. The colleagues in this case have fallen for a fixation error that was triggered by the symptoms (tachypnea) and the situation (typical environment and typical patient age for hyperventilation). If they had not let themselves be influenced by the situation and had not fixated on the obvious suspected diagnosis of "hyperventilation tetany", they would probably have noticed that the unconsciousness does not fit the situation. An algorithm for unconsciousness would have suggested a timely blood sugar test with a high probability. This would have made the problem of hyperglycemia noticeable earlier. However, the unconsciousness and not the tachypnea must be recognized as the leading problem. Therefore, the repeated critical re-evaluation is an important instrument to minimize such errors.

The medical industry often uses aviation as a model for error management because the culture of error is better developed there, for example through media-attracting accidents that generate corresponding pressure to act. By no means does everything run smoothly in aviation, there are also fixation errors there. A nice example is the flight of an Air Canada Boeing 767 that was supposed to fly from Montreal to Winnipeg in 1983. The cockpit crew calculated a mass of 22,283 from 12,589 liters in the tank and a weight of 1.77 pounds/liter—mathematically correct, but because the plane was calibrated in kilograms, the onboard computer assumed 22,283 kg of fuel. In fact, however, there were only 12,589 L $\times$ 0.803 kg/liter = 9144 kg of fuel in the tank, somewhat less than the imagined half. The cockpit crew recalculated several times, but did not recognize the error in the unit. In the end, the pilot said: "That's it, we're going". About halfway there was an engine failure due to fuel shortage and the plane was finally able to reach a retired military airfield in a glide, where the landing was made without injuries [5]. Here, too, the cockpit crew had fallen for a fixation error: Although the pilots felt that they had not tanked enough, the mathematical control always gave the same number despite several recalculations—that man and machine started from different units, they did not notice.

51.1 Conclusion

All alarms must be taken seriously, even if they appear to be nonsensical, implausible or bland, and we are unlikely to be able to tell great stories. Suspected diagnoses of the rescue control center or the first responders should always be critically questioned. You should also remain suspicious over time until all findings and the medical history "fit together" and are consistent. It is better to pay attention to findings that refute one's own thesis than to those that confirm this assumption.

References

1. Callaham M (1989) Hypoxic hazards of traditional paper bag rebreathing in hyperventilating patients. Ann Emerg Med 18:622–628
2. Baehner T, Heister U, Boehm O, Hoeft A, Knuefermann P (2012) Fixation errors in emergency medicine. Notfall Rettungsmedizin 15:606–611
3. Herrmann JM (1999) Series: functional disorders-functional breathing disorders. The hyperventilation syndrome. Dtsch Ärztebl Intl 96:694–697
4. Fioratou E, Flin R, Glavin R (2010) No simple fix for fixation errors: cognitive processes and their clinical applications. Anaesthesia 65:61–69
5. Richter JA (2008) Der Gimli Glider. Aerointernational 9:86–88

Hybrid-ECMO

52

Marc O. Maybauer

A 31-year-old patient, four months post-partum with a history of asthma, smoking and chronic back pain, was admitted to the emergency department of an outside hospital with the diagnosis of anaphylactic reaction. The first symptoms such as shortness of breath occurred after the initial administration of baclofen (a gamma aminobutyric acid derivate), which was prescribed to her for her lumbar pain syndrome. With a heart rate of 148/min, respiratory rate 38/min, blood pressure 127/101 mm Hg and an oxygen saturation of 89% on room air, she was initially given an oxygen mask at 4 l/min, epinephrine intramuscularly, as well as cortisone and an H1 antihistamine intravenously. She was admitted to the intensive care unit for monitoring. With increasing complaints, she was given a beta-2 sympathomimetic via nebulizer and BiPAP ventilation with light sedation was initiated. With increasing oxygen requirements, confusion and carbon dioxide retention, she was intubated and given nebulized epinephrine, which, however, did not alleviate the increasing bronchospasm. Sedation was then deepened with propofol. Over the next hours, despite ongoing therapy, a status asthmaticus developed with severe hypoxemia and hypercapnia. At this time, late in the evening of the day of admission, our "Shock & ECMO Center" was called and asked for help. About 45 min later, our ECMO team that had flown by helicopter, landed at the hospital, about 120 km (75 miles) away. By this time, the patient's condition, who was now in extremis with invasive ventilation (PIP 45 cmH$_2$O, PEEP 5 cmH$_2$O, FiO$_2$ 1.0), had deteriorated significantly. The arterial blood gas showed a pH of 6.9, PaO$_2$ 58 mmHg and a greatly increased, no longer measurable paCO$_2$ using a mobile blood gas analysis system. Clinically, there was a pronounced subcutaneous

M. O. Maybauer (✉)
University of Florida College of Medicine, Department of Anesthesiology,
Gainesville, Florida, USA
e-mail: mmaybauer@ufl.edu

© The Author(s), under exclusive license to Springer-Verlag GmbH, DE, part of Springer Nature 2023
V. Wenzel (ed.), *Case Studies in Emergency Medicine*,
https://doi.org/10.1007/978-3-662-67249-5_52

emphysema of the right chest, shoulder and neck region, which pointed to a pneumothorax. With this suspected diagnosis, we changed the sedation to ketamine/midazolam and paralyzed the patient with cis-atracurium, which unfortunately did not "resolve" the status asthmaticus. The chest X-ray taken in the meantime confirmed a tension pneumothorax; placement of a chest drain immediately led to an improvement in hemodynamics and reduction in norepinephrine infusion, but not to an improvement in oxygenation. Subsequently, a 25-Fr, 55 cm venous multistage ECMO cannula was inserted into the right femoral vein and a 23-Fr, 23 cm venous return cannula was inserted into the right internal jugular vein, and venovenous extracorporeal membrane oxygenation (V-V ECMO) and lung-protective ventilation were initiated. The $paCO_2$ was slowly lowered and by the time we arrived at our ECMO center, the patient already had normalized blood gases and was normotensive without the need for vasopressors. A transesophageal echocardiogram (TEE) was performed to exclude pericardial tamponade potentially due to ECMO cannulation and to document cardiac function, which showed a left ventricular ejection fraction (LVEF) of 70%. Thirty-six hours after ECMO cannulation the patient again developed hypotension and required high-dose norepinephrine. In the follow up TEE, the apical left ventricle was shown to be akinetic with an LVEF of about 20% and thus raised the suspicion of a stress-induced Takotsubo syndrome, which was confirmed by a relatively low troponin (1.29 ng/mL). With increasing lactic acidosis and vasopressor requirements, the V-V-ECMO configuration was extended to V-AV (veno-arteriovenous) in order to achieve respiratory and circulatory support. For this purpose, a 15-Fr cannula was placed in the left femoral artery, together with a 5 Fr antegrade distal perfusion cannula to optimize blood flow in this extremity. The blood flow from ECMO to the patient was now via a modified tubing system that distributed the return blood flow through a Y-piece to the vein and artery. Since the blood flow always follows the least resistance, only a blood flow of 1.5 l/min resulted in the arterial cannula (15-Fr) and about 4 l/min in the venous (23-Fr). This was unavoidable because the femoral artery of the rather delicate patient did not allow placement of a larger cannula due to its diameter. To compensate for this, we reduced the blood flow in the venous leg by partially clamping the tubing system and were able to generate a blood flow of about 2.5–3 l/min on both sides. This proved to be sufficient as the lactic acidosis gradually subsided. The following day, the LVEF was already in the range of 30%. However, the patient developed an MRSA-positive pneumonia, whereupon the prophylactic antibiotic therapy was changed from cefepime to vancomycin and ceftaroline. Due to the cardiogenic shock, the patient developed acute renal failure. The creatinine, which was 0.99 mg/dL at admission, rose to 3.1 mg/dL within four days, for which she received renal replacement therapy (CRRT). The daily echocardiogram showed an improvement in left ventricular function with an LVEF of 30–35%, 40–45% and 55–60% over the third, fourth and fifth day on V-AV ECMO. Now the arterial cannula, which was placed for circulatory support, could be removed, and the patient remained on respiratory support by V-V ECMO alone. On the right side, a complete collapse of the lung with a new tension pneumothorax developed over time, which led to the placement of another thoracic drainage.

In repeated bronchoscopies, purulent secretions could be suctioned from the lungs and a general improvement of the pulmonary situation could be achieved. On days 11 and 13, the blood cultures were negative for the first time. The collapsed lung could be recruited, and the patient was weaned from CRRT. On day 20, ECMO was explanted and the patient was transferred to the floor after 28 days in intensive care. After 40 days and rigorous physiotherapy, the patient was discharged home to her child "walking". This led to great joy of the entire team, which cared for this young mother very emotionally and selflessly during her hospital stay.

Discussion

This patient initially had a status asthmaticus with pneumothorax, caused by an anaphylactic reaction. Whether the pronounced hypoxemia and hypercapnia was exacerbated or caused by the development of an MRSA pneumonia and sepsis could not be demonstrated in the course of her hospital stay. The resulting severe stress reaction led to a Takotsubo syndrome with cardiogenic shock. The Takotsubo syndrome, which is caused by stress, leads to left ventricular failure due to endogenous catecholamine release, and is also described in association with infectious diseases and sepsis [1]. The Takotsubo syndrome can be treated with inotropic substances or V-A ECMO [2]. In our case, the diagnoses of anaphylaxis, refractory status asthmaticus, tension pneumothorax, MRSA pneumonia, sepsis and Takotsubo syndrome with cardiogenic shock could already cause a high morbidity / mortality rate by each comorbidity alone. The complex combination would have been fatal for this patient without ECMO. A recent meta-analysis [3] describes the technology change in the field of mechanical circulatory support (MCS) systems over the last decade with a significant reduction in the use of intra-aortic balloon pumps (IABP) compared to the Impella system and V-A ECMO, with V-A ECMO being used most frequently [3]. In our assessment, the IABP would have been of little use in this case, as it can only increase the pumping performance of the heart by an average of 10–15%. We were presented with the choice between Impella and V-A ECMO in the form of the V-AV configuration for left ventricular support, as V-V ECMO was already established. The implantation of a left ventricular assist device (LVAD) was not considered at this time, as the patient was hypoxemic and dependent on V-V ECMO. In our assessment, this was a probably reversible and short-term event for which V-A ECMO could be used as a temporary bridge to recovery [4]. During arterial cannulation, only a 15-Fr cannula was chosen due to the diameter of the femoral arteries. This is in contrast to our usual practice of using a 17-Fr cannula whenever possible. This unfortunately led to the above-mentioned problem of reduced blood flow, but this could be compensated for by partial clamping of the venous tubing system. A minimum of two l/min should flow through each cannula to reduce the risk of thrombus formation. After initiation of V-AV ECMO, the patient initially had borderline circulation and hypoxemia. When the venous side of the tubing system was clamped to increase the flow in the arterial leg, oxygenation worsened with improvement in hemodynamics and vice versa. Here, the ideal balance between oxygenation and circulatory support had to be found by repeatedly adjusting the clamp with different flow rates. At this point, we questioned our decision for V-A ECMO against Impella, as the Impella 5.0 or 5.5 could have generated higher flow rates. The Impella, which pumps blood out of the left ventricle into the aorta by means of an Archimedes' screw, shows good left ventricular unloading, especially with the high-flow devices such as Impella 5.0 or 5.5, while the devices (Impella 2.5 or CP) with flow rates of 2.5 to 3.5 l/min are less effective and are often used only to support V-A ECMO for left ventricular venting in case of insufficient contractility, as V-A ECMO results in a significant increase in afterload. The main advantage of ECMO is the possibility of oxygenation while providing circulatory support. The Impella should therefore only be used in patients with sufficient oxygenation in case of isolated cardiac pump failure. Since V-V ECMO already provided the possibility of oxygenation, an Impella 5.0/5.5 would have been a good alternative. In addition, the question arose as to central cannulation of the aorta, which, however, requires a sternotomy, which can cause additional complications and is considered obsolete in this case in the presence of peripheral MCS. At this point, we had found a setting of approximately 3 l/min each, which ensured oxygenation and slowly reduced the lactate level. Alternatively, the use of levosimendan, a calcium channel sensitizer, would have been possible to achieve inotropic support to reduce catecholamines. However, levosimendan is not currently approved by the US Food and Drug Administration, which is why we quickly dismissed this idea [5].

52.1 Conclusion

V-AV ECMO is a useful configuration for combined cardiorespiratory support. Benefits and risks must be weighed individually for each patient. The choice of cannula diameter and length should ideally be determined before implantation, although it is almost impossible to predict whether a patient will require a later change in configuration. The patient's age and optimal management by an experienced ECMO team, which treats approximately 150 ECMO patients per year, favored the therapeutic outcome. Patients with a similar pathology but higher Body Mass Index (BMI) are probably benefiting from the use of the Impella 5.0/5.5 to achieve sufficient blood flow and left ventricular unloading.

References

1. Li S, Koerner MM, El-Banayosy A, Soleimani B, Pae WE, Leuenberger UA (2014) Takotsubo's syndrome after mitral valve repair and rescue with extracorporeal membrane oxygenation. Ann Thorac Surg 97(5):1777–1778
2. De Giorgi A, Fabbian F, Pala M et al. (2015) Takotsubo cardiomyopathy and acute infectious diseases: a mini-review of case reports. Angiology 66(3):257–261
3. Mariani S, Richter J, Pappalardo F, et al. (2020) Mechanical circulatory support for Takotsubo syndrome: a systematic review and meta-analysis. Int J Cardiol Oct 1; 316:31–39.
4. Maybauer MO, El Banayosy A, Hooker RL et al. (2019) Percutaneous venoarterial extracorporeal membrane oxygenation as a bridge to double valve implantation in acute biventricular heart failure with profound cardiogenic shock. J Card Surg 34(12):1664–1666
5. Karvouniaris M, Papanikolaou J, Makris D, Zakynthinos E (2012) Sepsis-associated takotsubo cardiomyopathy can be reversed with levosimendan. Am J Emerg Med 30(5):832 e835–837.

Stop

53

Urs Pietsch

Just before the end of the day, we are called to a mountain biker who has fallen. Quickly, we sit in the EMS helicopter on the way to the site of the accident, which is about 15 min flight time away. We receive more detailed information about the injury during the flight by radio. We learn that a biker has overturned in a technically difficult descent and is now unconscious. We can get out of the helicopter and quickly reach the patient with our material while the helicopter can land a little lower. The patient presents with impaired A (airway) and B (breathing), probably as part of a severe head injury with a Glasgow Coma Scale of 6 points. The radial pulse is only weakly palpable. In addition, a laceration on the head and multiple bruises on the abdomen impress us at first glance. One of his friends reports that the injured person fell head first over the handlebars and remained motionless. While I am busy with the body check, my emergency medical technician has in the meantime inserted a large-volume intravenous access. We discuss the further treatment and its priorities as a team. The main problems are a severe head injury and a tense abdomen as a possible sign of liver or spleen laceration. We are in agreement: The patient must be intubated and quickly transported to a hospital of maximum care.

Although not ideal like in an ambulance, we are still in a suitable place for prehospital anesthesia induction and further treatment. We have access to the patient from all sides, an experienced team with emergency medical technician and emergency physician as well as additional help from the pilot and the patient's colleague, so we can treat the patient well. Drugs and materials are directed as well as another 10 for 10 (focused team time out) is carried out before laryngoscopy.

U. Pietsch (✉)
Department of Anesthesiology, Intensive Care, Emergency Medicine and Pain Therapy, Cantonal Hospital, St. Gallen, Switzerland
e-mail: Urs.Pietsch@kssg.ch

© The Author(s), under exclusive license to Springer-Verlag GmbH, DE, part of Springer Nature 2023
V. Wenzel (ed.), *Case Studies in Emergency Medicine*,
https://doi.org/10.1007/978-3-662-67249-5_53

Intubation is successful without problems. Afterwards, the patient is quickly evaluated from head to toe in the sense of a re-assessment. We quickly decide to inject 1 g of tranexamic acid in case of questionable intra-abdominal hemorrhage. We are satisfied with the condition of the patient, who is cardiopulmonally compensated by our therapy, and make our way towards the helicopter with the patient.

Then I relax next to the patient and sort all cables and tubes in the helicopter to get us ready for take-off. But what's blinking on the monitor? "Systole 60 mmHg"! Damn, what happened now? Do we now have a tension pneumothorax after intubation? Or did we underestimate the questionable intra-abdominal bleeding? Quickly the question is answered; instead of tranexamic acid, we grabbed the ampoule of the same size and color and injected it with the anitihypertensive drug Urapidil, an alpha-adrenoreceptorantagonist! How could this happen to us?

Discussion

Approximately 30–50% of all treatment errors are medication errors. Medication or dosage errors are among the most common errors in hospitals and outpatient clinics. For the USA, the literature assumes that 5% of all hospitalized patients experience a medication error every year; of these, 13% are serious. Professional societies and large hospital providers have now recognized the need for action to improve patient safety and have launched corresponding campaigns. A wide range of measures for better and more uniform labeling, mutual control, and standardized procedures for administration are intended to make the risks aware to employees and lead to a reduction in medication errors. Often, it is only after the injection of a medication that it is realized that an error has occurred; but then it is unfortunately too late because the medication is already in circulation. This is where one of the protection concepts comes in: all employees should take a short STOP just before injecting the medication (Stop-Inject Check!), then think about whether an error could occur so that it can still be corrected (Check!). The concept of the "Stop-Inject Check" only takes a few seconds, but can potentially reduce the error rate significantly [1]. Another established method for increasing safety and avoiding medication errors is the application of the so-called 5-R rule. Here, five questions are asked before each medication order and administration: Is it the right patient? The right medication? The right dosage? The right administration route and -location? The right time? The 4-eye principle—that is, showing the drawn-up medication including the ampoule—also contributes to safety. This re-check has nothing to do with mistrust of a given colleague. As in our case, it can happen quickly that the wrong ampoule is accidentally picked up. Very similar ampoule labels can quickly lead to unnoticed mix-ups; ampoules with similar appearances but different active ingredients should therefore under no circumstances be in the same corner of the emergency kit or anesthesia trolley. It can quickly become complicated if changing prices or delivery conditions lead to purchasing decisions in the pharmacy that abruptly negate these efforts. The statement "Said is not heard; heard is not understood and understood is not implemented" is of course also central to safe medication administration!

Standardized labels according to DIN ISO 26825 for drawn-up syringes enable a quick assignment of the medication group due to a color-coding and give the concentration in mg/ml again. If there are different blood vessel accesses, attention should also be paid to a color-coding in order to avoid accidental arterial drug injection. The labeling of venous (blue) and arterial (red) accesses by means of differently colored closure plugs and three-way stopcocks has established itself here.

In the described case, the classical error-favoring factors came together: the work environment with a high load directly after or during pre-hospital rapid sequence intubation in a severely injured patient, unclear responsibility in the team and individual factors, such as here the optically (size and label) very similar ampoules of Urapidil and Tranexamic acid [2]. In our described patient, hypotension caused by the injection of 50 mg Urapidil instead of 1 g Tranexamic acid could be quickly remedied by fractionated injection of noradrenaline. So it temporarily a potential vital danger of the patient developed, but fortunately no permanent damage occurred.

Each of us has already experienced such situations in which he was so sure that it is all but guaranteed not this. No, no, that's fine … Some things are so unimaginable that one does not believe it possible. But it can happen. For example, that laughing gas (N_2O) comes out of a ventilator instead of oxygen. In one case, anesthesia was initiated in a young man and a few minutes later he developed a cardiac arrest because anesthesia was induced with 100% N_2O and not 100% O_2 [3]. A lapidary ventilation with a self-inflating bag and room air would have solved the problem, but it was just unimaginable that something like this could happen. One was so fixated and so sure that it must be something else, but definitely not a problem with the ventilator. But during the setup of the workplace, the O_2 and N_2O lines were swapped and the device check or inspiratory gas measurement was ignored; in the end, a family father died unnecessarily. It was not the only case of accidental lethal N_2O ventilation—in a number of pregnant women with cardiac arrest in Germany, a placental embolism was suspected until a policeman simply locked the operating room because there was a death and an investigation was required. Otherwise, there might have been the next death because for health personnel a dead person on the operating table is nothing completely unimaginable, but for a policeman it is. Only if one discusses such a scenario of accidental swapped gas lines outside the immediate workplace, one has the chance to prevent it later [4].

Such fixation errors meet us very often in clinical everyday life and they represent one of the main reasons for incidents in the medical field. In complex situations, we can, for example, get so involved in administering a given activity that we do not even realize that much more important things are being forgotten or misinterpreted in the process [5]. This becomes quite drastic, for example, as in our case, when we are so fixated on one thing and so sure that we have taken the right ampoule that we totally lose sight of normal procedures (read the label without stress, 5-R-rule and stop-check-inject again). This becomes even more clear with manual and mentally demanding activities, such as difficult intubation. Quickly, one no longer perceives anything around oneself and is trapped in one's tunnel vision. A good, but tragic example of this is the case of Elaine Bromily in England [6]. The patient died during routine surgery because the anesthesia nurses correctly assessed the "can not intubate can not ventilate" situation and handed over a coniotomy set, which the experienced anesthetists did not want to use. In clinical everyday life, we are most often exposed to the risk of such fixation during diagnosis. Thoughts like; "This—and only this—it is"… "Everything but not that one it is"… "It's all right"… often lead to this fixation dead end. A constant and honest re-evaluation in the team is usually a successful strategy to avoid these fixation errors and to break free from them again.

53.1 Conclusion

The work environment of emergency medicine is particularly error-prone because composition of the teams and the work environment often change. Often, prehospital care is provided under unfavorable conditions for patients at risk of life, which automatically creates a high level of expectation and action pressure on the treatment team, which in turn can lead to errors. Simple thought supports such as the "stop-inject-check", 5-R-rule or uniform "labeling" can be helpful to prevent avoidable errors.

References

1. Koppenberg J, Henninger M, Gausmann P, Rall M (2011) Patient safety in emergency services: what contribution can CRM and teamwork make? Der Notarzt 27:249–254. https://doi.org/10.1055/s-0031-1276905
2. Pierre St, Hofinger G (2020) Human Factors and Patient Safety in Acute Care, 3rd edition ISBN 978–3–642–55420–9
3. Herff H, Paal P, Lindner K et al (2008) Nitrous oxide related deaths. Anaesthesist 57:1006. https://doi.org/10.1007/s00101-008-1434-7
4. Herff H, Paal P, von Goedecke A, Lindner KH, Keller C, Wenzel V (2007) Fatal errors in nitrous oxide delivery. Anaesthesia 62(12):1202–1206. https://doi.org/10.1111/j.1365-2044.2007.05193.x PMID: 17991254
5. Singh JM, MacDonald RD, Bronskill SE, Schull MJ (2009) Incidence and predictors of critical events during urgent air-medical transport. CMAJ 181(9):579–584. https://doi.org/10.1503/cmaj.080886
6. https://www.youtube.com/watch?v=44tH98eLrkQ. Accessed 18 Feb 2021

54

Urs Pietsch

It is one of those beautiful autumn days in the mountains. We sit relaxed in front of the hangar in the sun and enjoy the silence. In this time, between the winter and the summer high season, it is often quiet here in the mountains, while in the high season the scene calls follow one after the other. Then a crashed hiker in a remote mountain valley pulls us out of the midday break. Quickly we sit in the EMS helicopter and fly in the direction of the reported accident site. Over the radio we learn that a hiker from a group of five people has stumbled and fallen down a steep slope. The group had called several times for the person, but had received no answer. I go through possible scenarios: How severe is the trauma, is a landing possible, how dangerous is the terrain, which target hospital could be suitable, how is the weather … While I am thinking, we are already hovering above the reported position. Quickly the group of hikers is spotted from the air. But where is the patient? About 100 altitude meters or 330 feet below, a person is located lifeless between the rocks. A landing here is impossible, so I will be lowered to the patient with the rescue winch. My paramedic stays in the helicopter as a winch operator. So I float alone with a physician's bag and a mountain bag (including a vacuum mattress for rescuing of the patient by winch) to the patient. Once I arrive at the bottom, it quickly becomes clear that the patient is seriously injured but still alive. An irregular, gurgling respiration quickly points to a severe head injury together with an enlarged pupil. "Everything is fine," I think to myself, "A and B have to be secured, so an intubation!" Quickly I put on a pulse oximeter, the oxygen saturation is only 73% at a heart rate of 65/min. Confirmed by these values, I further arrange the drugs, the laryngoscope and the tube for a rapid sequence

U. Pietsch (✉)
Department of Anesthesiology, Intensive Care, Emergency Medicine and Pain Therapy, Cantonal Hospital, St. Gallen, Switzerland
e-mail: Urs.Pietsch@kssg.ch

V. Wenzel (ed.), *Case Studies in Emergency Medicine*,
https://doi.org/10.1007/978-3-662-67249-5_54

intubation and insert an intravenous access. To be honest, it really doesn't work quickly. Arranging material alone and without additional help and looking after the patient at the same time, let alone storing it in the mountain bag for transport, takes time. "When are you ready to be picked up?" Sounds through the radio and pulls me out of my world. Is it really clever and realistic what I am doing here? This cannot be done alone, let alone safely cared for. "In five minutes you can pick me up, please prepare everything for an intubation at the intermediate loading point!" I report back. Quickly I pack all the arranged things into the doctor's bag, store the patient as best I can in the stable side position and with a Guedel tube to keep the airways open in the mountain bag and get ready for the winch action. A few minutes later, the patient and I float together on the winch under the helicopter hanging over the valley towards the intermediate landing point. Together, in a well-rehearsed team, the patient is intubated and prepared for transport to the hospital.

Discussion

The case described here shows important aspects of alpine emergency medicine. Often, missions are carried out as in tactical medicine and "care under fire", namely in a difficult environment. Wind, cold, darkness or strong sunlight in the snow, in addition limited working conditions or even dangerous terrain limit the possibilities of care and force us to plan our actions deliberately and foreseeingly and to deviate from guideline-conform algorithms. In the case described, it is clear to all colleagues active in emergency medicine that airway management in the event of a head injury and as a result of impaired protective reflexes and insufficient respiration has high priority. Together in a well-rehearsed team in an ambulance, this rarely poses a problem. In mountain rescue, one often works alone, because the paramedic remains as a winch operator in the EMS helicopter, or also in randomly composed teams. These ad-hoc teams consist, for example, of mountain rescue specialists or ski slope rescuers who have very different medical skills [1–4]. In addition, they are often little or completely unknown to us, with whom we have no routine in cooperation, including all the resulting problems.

In principle, simple measures, such as drawing up drugs, setting up an infusion, an endotracheal tube or the optimal positioning of a patient, are partly significantly more difficult or even impossible in the alpine environment and under adverse conditions. So at significant minus degrees a syringe or infusion is quickly frozen and drugs can not be applied at all. The downwash of the helicopter reliably blows away any perfectly directed material. Intubation alone or before winch rescue is also technically possible in alpine terrain, but requires a very critical risk-benefit assessment. What use is a formally secured airway if I can not ensure continuous ventilation, or if there is a tube dislocation during the rescue mission or during the winch operation?

If you use an invasive measure, you can stabilize an unstable situation or turn an unstable situation into a catastrophe. We have all experienced it before, that, for example, a too young operating room team initiates a too large surgical procedure on a too unstable patient too late at night and afterwards nothing was as it was before. Although you will hardly find descriptions of these cases in the literature, this is probably the "negative publication bias", that you simply omit publishing certain unpleasant things. On the other hand, you don't have to look long in the literature to find reports of intubation errors. The incidence of unrecognized pre-hospital intubation errors is better in German-speaking countries than in the USA, but of course still associated with high mortality [5]. The regular use of capnography to control a correct endotracheal intubation has had a positive impact on faster and safer control of correct intubation in recent years and also offers the EMS team an objective parameter in hectic situations to quickly recognize and correct a potential intubation error. In addition, technical developments in recent years, such as the now widespread use of video laryngoscopy, aim to increase the so-called First Pass Success (intubation on the first attempt). In experienced hands, this has led to an improvement in the First Pass Success. However, all these aids should not lead to a false sense of security of the team on site and make the respect for difficult airway situations disappear. Various publications have shown that, for example, due to the problem of the partly good visualization of the vocal cord level by means of video laryngoscopy, but an impossibility of the correct tracheal positioning of the tube, more desaturations and relevant hypoxemia could be detected than by means of classical laryngoscopy. This underlines how important training and education for all colleagues working in emergency medicine is, despite technology. Not only technical skills are essential, but also the handling of human factors and human errors.

Anesthesiologists like to make fun of non-Anesthesiologists who "cannot intubate", but at the same time create pressure to intubate by making casual comments in the emergency room like "Why doesn't the patient come to us intubated?" It is logical that in such a case a non-Anesthesiologist initiates intubation pre-hospitally, but the situation is more difficult than expected or his own experience and pharmacological strategy is not as good as expected and the situation gets out of control. In the emergency room I have almost never experienced that a non-Anesthesiologist said: "The situation was too dangerous for me outside; therefore I did not initiate any invasive airway management in order to control it later in the emergency room with more personnel, experience and better conditions." This decision is the smartest of all—whoever knows and communicates his own limits, his team and his material can save lives by (almost) not doing anything (for example, Wendl/Guedel tube in spontaneous respiration instead of anesthesia initiation with subsequent "cannot intubate cannot ventilate" scenario) [6].

54.1 Conclusion

In mountain rescue, whether terrestrial or air-based, it often requires deviating from established supply concepts. Environmental conditions dictate the extent and sequence of measures that are useful on site and which should follow at a later time. Ad-hoc teams assembled are an additional challenge in this environment. This problem and the associated problems are also transferable to the entire emergency medicine. Special requirements must be trained beforehand to ensure a safe supply for both the patient and the rescuer. Less can be more quickly, as the right intervention in the wrong place or at the wrong time can go wrong quickly. Knowing your own limits, those of the team and of the material and communicating them openly is particularly important in emergency medicine for a safe patient care.

References

1. Pietsch U, Knapp J, Kreuzer O, Ney L, Strapazzon G, Lischke V et al (2018) Advanced airway management in hoist and longline operations in mountain HEMS – considerations in austere environments: a narrative review this review is endorsed by the International Commission for Mountain Emergency Medicine (ICAR MEDCOM). Scand J Trauma Resusc Emerg Med. 26(1):23
2. Lischke V, Berner A, Pietsch U, Schiffer J, Ney L (2014) Medical simulation training of helicopter-supported mountain rescue situations (MedSim-BWZSA). Notfall Rettungsmed. 2012(17):46–52
3. Pietsch U, Ney L, Kreuzer O, Berner A, Lischke V (2017) Helicopter emergency medical service simulation training in the extreme: simulation-based training in a mountain weather chamber. Air Med J 36(4):193–194
4. Pietsch U, Strapazzon G, Ambühl D et al (2019) Challenges of helicopter mountain rescue missions by human external cargo: need for physicians onsite and comprehensive training. Scand J Trauma Resusc Emerg Med 27:17. https://doi.org/10.1186/s13049-019-0598-2
5. Timmermann A, Russo SG, Eich C, Roessler M, Braun U, Rosenblatt WH, Quintel M (2007) The out-of-hospital esophageal and endobronchial intubations performed by emergency physicians. Anesth Analg 104(3):619–623. https://doi.org/10.1213/01.ane.0000253523.80050.e9
6. von Goedecke A, Keller C, Voelckel WG et al (2006) Maskenbeatmung als Rückzugsstrategie zur endotrachealen Intubation. Anaesthesist 55:70–79. https://doi.org/10.1007/s00101-005-0927-x

Quiet Voice

Sylvi Thierbach

February 2015, Mazar-e-Sharif, Afghanistan. Our German field hospital is set up like a small district hospital for the treatment of our own and allied soldiers: surgery, anesthesia, internal medicine, radiology with a CT, six intensive care beds, a small ward, emergency department, laboratory, two operating rooms, sterilization, a dental unit and a general practitioner; a total of 50 people. It's a relatively quiet time. There are few attacks or fighting probably due to the cold, unpleasant weather—in the field hospital normal operation is running and there are no patients in the intensive care unit. In the afternoon we receive the request to treat in our field hospital a small Afghan girl with head and brain trauma after a collision with a car. At the beginning of the mission in Afghanistan, the treatment of civilians under the motto "winning hearts and minds" was favored and took place regularly. During the course of the military operation, this changed and the treatment of Afghan civilians required approval of the military leadership. Fortunately, the decision to treat the girl was granted quickly. However, it should be noted that the current calm situation could change quickly with an immediate need for intensive care beds. But there is hardly any alternative for the girl in this place. A land-based transfer to the nearest children's hospital in Kabul would take a day or more for the 430 km (267 miles) due to the bad road conditions over the Hindukush mountains and an airlift would not be available. Although emergency equipment for children is available, we do not have a stock of consumables for long-term treatment, as this is not the primary task of the field hospital.

Four hours after the initial call, 4-year-old Farzana arrives at the field hospital in an ambulance with a red crescent. At first glance, the prognosis is not

S. Thierbach (✉)
Federal Armed Forces Hospital, Department of Anesthesiology, Intensive Care, Emergency Medicine and Pain Therapy, Ulm, Germany
e-mail: s.maget@hamburg.de

V. Wenzel (ed.), *Case Studies in Emergency Medicine*,
https://doi.org/10.1007/978-3-662-67249-5_55

good—although Farzana is breathing spontaneously with a nasogastric tube and is hemodynamically stable, her Glasgow Coma Scale is only 6, her pupils react isocoric and only sluggish to light; she vomits when turned. We intubate immediately and perform a CT, which shows a covered head trauma with a small intracranial bleed, but thankfully no brain edema. Neurosurgical colleagues in Germany confirm the diagnosis by telemedicine; there is no indication for surgical intervention and we transfer Farzana to the intensive care unit. In the coming days, pediatric intensivists from our own circle of friends in Germany become our telephone jokers—we discuss findings, sedation and nutrition regimes, and after a few days we are able to extubate Farzana without problems. At first we are optimistic, but neurologically she does not show any progress in the following days. Although she has protective reflexes, she has synergistic flexion and does not fixate, her Glasgow Coma Scale is borderline, so that we discuss re-intubation on a daily basis. Many employees of the field hospital spend hours at Farzana's bedside, read to her and help her with physiotherapy and occupational therapy. Almost every day, her father and her cousin Farzana visit, but their efforts in familiar language do not change the condition of our little patient. After another two weeks, our relief arrives. We are allowed to go home. Actually a moment that you look forward to after being two months abroad, but we travel home with a heavy heart and mixed feelings. What will become of Farzana?

We stay in close contact with our successors and are pleased to hear that Farzana is becoming more awake, starting to fixate and eat, that even bed rails are needed, which have to be made specially by the employees of the field hospital, and now prevent the increasingly mobile Farzana from tumbling out of the big bed. One day we receive a voice message and with tears in our eyes we hear Farzana's soft voice trying to imitate the colleagues. It was the "toughest" men who were moved the most. Farzana can finally be discharged from the field hospital after a total of six weeks of treatment. Three years later I am back in that field hospital in Mazar-e-Sharif, and after long efforts by the special forces and their contacts, who have to find the girl's father with great difficulty, I see her again. She goes to school, learns to read and write. She is shy, but an alert child and the parents are overjoyed that their daughter has been given a chance at a good life in a society in which women have hardly any rights and medical care is only rudimentary in large parts of the country.

Discussion

Child emergencies are and remain situations for all those who work in emergency medicine, which one approaches with great respect. In the injured or seriously ill children one sees possibly one's own child and is automatically affected. The concern increases when we come across child emergencies in an environment in which we cannot draw on full medical resources and the lack of resources can impose a limitation of therapy. In Afghanistan, according to data from the WHO [6, 7 and 8], medical care of the civilian population is precarious due to the ongoing war for over 40 years with only few interruptions. In 2015, there were only three physicians and three nurses/midwives and four hospital beds per 10,000 inhabitants in Kabul. In Germany, there are almost 12 times as many doctors and 20 times as many hospital beds per inhabitant. Many medical facilities in Afghanistan are poorly equipped, there is a lack of specialist personnel and the security situation leads again and again to destruction and closures. Although medical care is free of charge in state hospitals in Afghanistan, the costs of hospitalization, required medication, examinations and treatment must usually be paid for by the family. The family also takes care of the patient in the hospital [2]. Many Afghan families cannot afford such medical care or do not have access to medical care facilities of a higher level in urban areas due to a rural location. Rehabilitation facilities, such as those we know in Germany, for example, for follow-up care in the event of a severe head injury, and which are available in sufficient numbers, are completely lacking.

In crisis areas, children make up a significant proportion of patients requiring treatment [5]. Approximately 10% of patients receiving medical intervention in military facilities in crisis areas such as Iraq or Afghanistan were children with an average age of approximately 12 years [3, 4]. As military physicians, we regularly treat children in emergency medicine and in everyday operating room practice at home in German Armed Forces hospitals, although not as frequently as our civilian colleagues in children's hospitals. However, German Armed Forces hospitals are not designed for intensive care of children, so routine care is lacking here. This makes the possibility of telemedicine all the more important for us, which has not yet been established in Germany due to many uncertainties, such as incompatible IT interfaces and standards, lack of acceptance, data protection problems, and unresolved legal framework conditions [1]. In our case, telemedicine in radiological diagnostics with radiologists and neurosurgeons alike represented a relevant and essential gain in information and professional exchange, and in terms of intensive care for children, it offered better patient safety through professional exchange. Admission and treatment of the girl in a facility equipped with material and personnel according to Western standards meant a real chance of survival, which would otherwise have been very likely to be close to zero due to the medical treatment situation described above in Afghanistan.

55.1 Conclusion

Thanks to the entire medical team of the field hospital and our friendly colleagues in intensive care for children in Germany, we were able to make a decisive difference for the child and her family in the case of Farzana. Cases like this bring treatment teams together and will also continue to provide special interdisciplinary cohesion in German Armed Forces hospitals in the future, far beyond the deployment period. Those who have worked together far beyond their comfort zone will function together in the interests of the patient and the team at home even better. It is precisely these experiences and the shared sense of success that make these deployments so valuable to us, despite the recurrent absences from home, from family and friends.

References

1. R Klar, E Pelikan (2009) State, possibilities and limitations of telemedicine in Germany. Bundesgesundheitsblatt – Gesundheitsforschung – Gesundheitsschutz 52(3):263–269
2. Korzilius H (2008) The principle of hope, medical care in Afghanistan. Dtsch Arztebl 105:A-267
3. Mauer UM, Freude G, Schulz C, Kunz U, Mathieu R (2017) Pediatric Neurosurgical Care in a German Field Hospital in Afghanistan. J Neurol Surg A Cent Eur Neurosurg 78(1):20–24
4. Naylor JF, April MD, Roper JL, Hill GJ, Clark P, Schauer SG (2018) Emergency department imaging of pediatric trauma patients during combat operations in Iraq and Afghanistan. Pediatr Radiol 48(5):620–625
5. Pannell D, Poynter J, Wales P W, Tien H, Nathens A B, Shellington D (2015) Factors affecting mortality of pediatric trauma patients encountered in Kandahar, Afghanistan; Can J Surg, 58:141–145
6. http://www.emro.who.int/images/stories/afghanistan/who_at_a_glance_2019_feb.pdf?ua=1. Accessed 2 Jan 2021
7. http://www.emro.who.int/images/stories/afghanistan/joint_country_programme_j_afghanistan_2018_2019.pdf?ua=1. Accessed 2 Feb 2021
8. http://www.ippnw.de/commonFiles/pdfs/Frieden/Akt21_Afghanistan.pdf. Accessed 2 Jan 2021

Quarantine

56

Petra Tietze-Schnur

The Sunday before Christmas, a physician-manned ambulance is deployed early in the morning with the message: "lifeless person". When we arrived, the patient's husband greeted us and led us into the garden. There we find the hanged wife of the man; she is not even 50 years old. She has lividity and of course asystole; we stop the chest compressions started by the first responder. The husband tells us that his wife had a positive Corona virus test ten days ago, but no disease symptoms; she was therefore in home quarantine. For a few days, according to the husband, she had increasingly "strange" symptoms—she had delusions of her person and was of the opinion that "our water, land and soil are contaminated", "how can one ever get that clean again". The husband asked me: "Why did she do that?", But I had no answer. The husband reported that he had been worried and contacted the family physician non-emergency service hotline the day before. There he was told that the EMS was responsible. He then chose the EMS emergency number, described his problem and received the statement that "the EMS is not responsible for that". Then there was a longer conversation with a local chaplain in the evening, which is said to have calmed the wife down a bit. In the morning the husband got up (they had separate bedrooms because of the quarantine) and wondered that his wife was not in the kitchen as usual. Since the door to the garden was open, he looked and found his wife lifeless.

P. Tietze-Schnur (✉)
Day Clinic at the Ocean, Bremerhaven, Germany
e-mail: pts@anaesthesie-am-meer.de

Discussion

The Spanish flu pandemic (1918–1920; worldwide about 30–50 million deaths, including more than 400,000 in the then German Reich) caused an increase in suicide rates, which was probably due to fears of the pandemic and reduced social integration. In our time, the Corona epidemic is an unimaginable social, economic, political and health crisis for all of us, exposing each of us to an unimaginable stress. Scientists at the University of Kentucky even describe the Corona circumstances as a "perfect storm" that destabilizes vulnerable people and thus increases the risk of suicide: an intensification of social isolation through lockdown measures, economic difficulties due to short-time work, unemployment or collapse of entire industries, difficult access to outpatient medical care, unlimited sale of alcohol, ban on public leisure activities such as swimming pool, gym, restaurants, libraries, etc., double burdens through home office and home schooling as well as relationship problems in the family and partnerships [1]. In the USA, the problem is compounded by the fact that there are 396 million firearms in private hands for a population of 326 million [2], which practically anyone can use to commit suicide with a firearm at any time if all the fuses "blow". Nine of the ten weeks with the highest number of requests for a background check for a gun purchase from the US federal police FBI since 1998 have been since the beginning of the pandemic 2020 [3]. One victim was a 24-year-old man in Traverse City, Michigan with depression and anxiety disorders; his therapist had to close his practice, his college too, his father lost his job, his mother tried desperately to find a therapy place for her son within a radius of 1500 km (932 miles) but always ended up on answering machines. The mother finally found a note on his desk: "I am sorry. I love you all". Almost all shops were closed, but not the gun shop, where he bought a gun for 560.67 US$ and shot himself in a park. Before official national statistics are available on whether suicides have become more frequent during the coronavirus pandemic, it will take one to two years. Significant regional increases of around 25% have been reported, for example, in Arizona, Oregon, Chicago and Japan. For example, a father found notes from his son after his son's suicide during the coronavirus pandemic about how much he missed meeting his three best friends, who had helped him through difficult phases of his depression. Studies show that even simple personal care by concerned friends or family members during such an apparently unstable phase can significantly reduce the suicide rate or a carefully taking medical history making paramedics or admitting physicians in the hospital who identify suicidal thoughts and initiate the appropriate consultations or treatment [4].

The personal despair caused by the coronavirus pandemic continues in other cases worldwide with suicides. In Lockport, Illinois/USA, in April 2020, a 54-year-old shot his 59-year-old girlfriend, who was suffering from severe breathing problems; he then shot himself. He was afraid that he had contracted the coronavirus from his girlfriend. Both had taken a coronavirus test, but had not learned the result before their death. The autopsy showed that neither of them was infected with the coronavirus [5]. In Amritsar, India, in April 2020, a 65-year-old man and his wife committed suicide with an oral poison. They left a farewell letter in which they wrote: "We are ending our lives. No one is responsible for this. There was great pressure because of Covid-19. We were also sick." [6]. In April 2020, a young couple committed suicide in Uttarakand, India, a few months after their wedding. The man was in quarantine without any Covid-19 symptoms outside his home village; his wife was pressured by neighbors to leave the village because they thought her husband was Covid-19 positive. She then visited her husband and the couple saw the situation as so hopeless that they hanged themselves from a tree; shortly before, they communicated this via WhatsApp to their home village [7]. In May 2020, a couple in Bihar, India, was unable to service a loan for a delivery van because they had no work because of Covid-19. The woman burned herself and died in the hospital; her husband then hanged himself. The couple left two children (7 and 10 years old) [2]. At the end of March, a 49-year-old nurse had agreed to work on the new Covid-19 in Jesolo, Italy. She got a fever, took a coronavirus test, and was then alone at home; shortly afterwards, she jumped from a bridge into a river and drowned. The test result remained unknown. In London, England, at the end of March 2020, a young nurse was found dead on the intensive care unit. Eight patients on this intensive care unit had died shortly before, there was a shortage of staff and personal protective equipment. Also at the end of March, a 34-year-old nurse was tested positive for the coronavirus on an intensive care unit in a suburb of Milan, Italy. She was stressed by the terrible events in this region, which was extremely hard hit by the Covid-19 pandemic, and committed suicide in her quarantine. In May 2020, a 32-year-old nurse worked voluntarily on a Corona unit in Florida. He was very worried about a shortage of personal protective equipment and developed strong fears and trauma. He was supported by digital meetings; the day before his suicide, the digital meeting was canceled and he felt secretions on his face when intubating [8]. At the end of April 2020, the medical director of an emergency room in New York City told her family about terrible impressions of Covid-19 patients. Later she became infected with Corona at work, went into quarantine, returned to work too early, was sent home again, and then visited her family in the neighboring state, where she committed suicide [9]. Her father said: "She tried to do her job, and it killed her."

It is relatively easy to say that the risk of "corona suicides" can be reduced by reducing stress, anxiety, and loneliness. People must be encouraged to sleep enough, eat healthy, talk about their fears and concerns, and not neglect physical activity on traditional ways and if this is not possible digitally through family, friends, and media [10]. The Corona crisis is likely to generate a breakthrough in telemedicine because consultations are possible in a low-threshold and geographically independent manner. Although this was already technically possible before Covid-19, it was avoided for a variety of reasons. If help is needed, this can be done at any time in a low-threshold manner via telefonseelsorge.de in Germany, telefonseelsorge.at in Austria or the Dargebotene Hand (143. ch) in Switzerland.

56.1 Conclusion

The risk of suicide during the coronavirus pandemic is probably increased in people who already have mental health problems, for example, due to social isolation, economic difficulties, and difficult access to therapists and leisure activities. Detailed official statistics are not yet available. Dispatchers in rescue control centers as well as EMS personnel and emergency physicians at the scene should question any unclear situation in patients with potential suicidal thoughts as long as necessary, research, organize, and treat until a satisfactory solution or treatment has been found for all involved.

References

1. Brown S, Schumann DL (2021) Suicide in the time of COVID-19: A perfect storm. J Rural Health 37:211–214
2. https://www.washingtonpost.com/news/wonk/wp/2018/06/19/there-are-more-guns-than-people-in-the-united-states-according-to-a-new-study-of-global-firearm-ownership/. Accessed 1 Jan 2021
3. https://www.fbi.gov/file-repository/nics_firearm_checks_top_10_highest_days_weeks.pdf/view. Accessed 1 Jan 2021
4. https://www.washingtonpost.com/health/2020/11/23/covid-pandemic-rise-suicides/. Accessed 8 Feb 2021
5. https://www.bbc.com/news/world-us-canada-52192842. Accessed 31 Dec 2020
6. Griffiths MD, Mamun MA (2020) COVID-19 suicidal behavior among couples and suicide pacts: case study evidence from press reports. Psychiatry Res 289:113105
7. https://www.telegraphindia.com/india/hounded-over-coronaviruscouple-%20%20kill-themselves/cid/1765526. Accessed 31 Dec 2020
8. Rahman A, Plummer V (2020) COVID-19 related suicide among hospital nurses; case study evidence from worldwide media reports. Psychiatry Res 291:113272
9. https://www.nytimes.com/2020/04/27/nyregion/new-york-city-doctor-suicide-coronavirus.html. Accessed 31 Dec 2020
10. Sher L (2020) The impact of COVID-19 on suicide rates. QJM 113:707–712